PARASITES AND PARASITIC DISEASES

RECENT ADVANCES IN TOXOPLASMOSIS RESEARCH

Parasites and Parasitic Diseases

Additional books in this series can be found on Nova's website under the Series tab.

Additional e-books in this series can be found on Nova's website under the e-book tab.

PARASITES AND PARASITIC DISEASES

RECENT ADVANCES IN TOXOPLASMOSIS RESEARCH

CONNOR M. LEE
EDITOR

New York

Library of Congress Cataloging-in-Publication Data

ISBN: 978-1-63117-914-3
LCCN: 2014938432

Published by Nova Science Publishers, Inc. † New York

CONTENTS

PREFACE

Toxoplasmosis is one of the most important foodborne illnesses and fetal maternal inflammatory syndromes. Currently, there is no safe and effective approved therapy against fetal maternal complication or persistent chronic infection. Toxoplasma is an intracellular organism. About 1.5 billion people worldwide are predicted to have toxoplasmosis, frequently with unknown lifelong health consequences. Toxoplasma is classified as "Category B pathogen" according to the Center for Disease Control (CDC) and National Institute of Health (NIH). The organisms reside in muscles and brain in cyst forms for the lifetime of the host awaiting reactivation. This book discusses several topics which include fetal and maternal toxoplasmosis; toxoplasma gondii and suicide and homicide; toxoplasmosis in several animals including cattle, goats, swine, dogs, and kittens; and molecular diagnosis in toxoplasmosis.

Chapter 1 - Toxoplasmosis is one of the most important foodborne illness and fetal maternal inflammatory syndromes. Currently, there is no safe and effective approved therapy against fetal maternal complication or persistent chronic infection. *Toxoplasma* has a sexual stage in intestinal epithelia of the cats, to form resistant oocysts. A predominant source of human infection in North America is considered to be contaminated food and water with oocysts rather than cysts forms. Fetus becomes infected by transplacental transmission acquired from infected mom with an acute or the reactivation of the chronic or latent infection due to the stressors during pregnancy. *Toxoplasma* invades fetal central nervous system with adverse affect in brain neuro-structural development and pathological as well as psycho-behavioral alteration leading to mental retardation. T*oxoplasma* has a unique mind/brain altering effect with increased sexual attractions and is a sexually transmissible disease through contaminated semen. In this chapter, fetal maternal toxoplasmosis, complication, diagnosis, current therapies and a novel anti-fetal maternal toxoplasmosis therapy is discussed with a promising future for clinical trial.

Chapter 2 - Studies of European nations have found that the prevalence of the brain parasite *Toxoplasma gondii* is positively associated with both suicide and homicide rates. In addition, research on individuals has shown that the presence of *T. gondii* is associated with fatal and non-fatal suicidal behavior in both men and women. The mediating physiological processes for these associations may involve the neurotransmitter dopamine, the amino acid tryptophan and the hormone testosterone, all of which are impacted by the presence of *T. gondii.*

Chapter 3 - Bovines acquire Toxoplasma gondii mainly by congenital route and by ingestion of food or water containing oocysts, and soil contaminated with cat manure. These animals may be relatively resistant to infection, since the detection of cysts in their musculature is less frequent than in other species, despite being evidenced high occurrence of the parasite in serological surveys. In bovine the main means of prevention is the correct storage of food and water without contact with the feces of cats. Humans are infected mainly by eating raw or undercooked bovine meat as well by ingestion of not pasteurized or boiled milk. Prophylaxis for a human being is to avoid the consumption of raw animal foods must be processed by baking, boiling or freezing, and the parasite is responsive to three if performed appropriately. In this context, new worldwide perspectives referring to means of transmission, clinical signs, diagnosis and treatments in cattle will be discussed.

Chapter 4 - *Toxoplasma gondii* is the etiologic agent of a worldwide distribution zoonosis. Cats are denominated as definitive hosts, but the infection affects many species including goats. Ingestion of oocysts excreted in definitive hosts feces, as well as water and soil, and via the transplacental represents the source of contamination. Goats infected with *T. gondii* will develop fever, anorexia, dyspnea, and pregnant females, in addition to those mentioned signs, will suffer miscarriage and stillbirth. Therefore this chapter will discuss relevant topics on the epidemiology, clinical signs, diagnosis, treatment and control of this disease so important and widespread in the world.

Chapter 5 - Toxoplasmosis is a cosmopolitan zoonosis transmitted primarily by cats infected with the protozoan. It affects human and several other species including swine. The species merits special attention because it is considered by epidemiologists an important reservoir and source of infection to human populations due to the longevity of tissue cysts. The prevalence of swine toxoplasmosis can vary greatly according to the socio-cultural habits, geographical and climatic factors. In this chapter the authors discuss the seroprevalence of *Toxoplasma gondii* in swines, epidemiological data, even as immunologic reactions of organic animal front ace infections, the main forms of diagnosis used and the possible advances that can contribute to the prevention of these animals.

Chapter 6 - Toxoplamosis is considered major parasitary disease in sheep, due its importance in veterinary medicine and animal science and in public health. In ewe the main clinical repercussion is abortion, economic losses through embryonic and fetal death, still birth and neonatal losses, represents an obstacle in profitability in worldwide sheep farm production. Amongst food producing animals, sheep meat was considered to be highest risk food for transmission of toxoplasmosis to humans, furthermore recent studies have been found cases of excretion of the parasite from milk of naturally infected sheep, suggesting a potential source of infection to humans when consumed without prior boiling or pasteurization, which can facilitate the zoonotic transmission. New research has shown that repeat ovine transmission of *T. gondii* in subsequent pregnancies can occur, unlike previous studies suggest that sheep have aborted due to parasite develop protection against future abortion. In these animals is likely that reactivation of latent toxoplasmosis can occur and influence the high incidence of infection in sheep. The main objective of this chapter will be discussing important aspects involving new advances in the epidemiology, diagnosis and control of this important disease in sheep industry.

Chapter 7 - The protozoan parasite *Toxoplasma gondii* commonly infects cats, dogs and humans. Toxoplasmosis is an important issue concerning public health, particularly involving the risk of disease transmission during pregnancy. The infection can be acquired by ingestion of tissue cysts in infected meat, ingestion of food or water contaminated with oocysts and congenitally, by tachyzoites crossing the placenta from the infected mother to the fetus. Congenital *T. gondii* infection has been reported in many species of animals. The organism strain, dose, and the stage of fetal development or age of the host at the time of infection likely influence the presence or severity of clinical toxoplasmosis in the neonate. The infecting stage of the organism (tachyzoite, oocyst, cyst) may also be important. Uterine changes were observed in bitches with toxoplasmosis (endometritis). Cats with disseminated organism replication which in clinical toxoplasmosis usually have multiple organ involvement that commonly includes the eyes. Ocular toxoplasmosis can occur without other evidence of clinical illness in kittens infected in uterus or in the neonatal period, and *T. gondii* strains may have varying degrees of ocular pathogenicity in cats. The aim of this chapter will be to elucidate some clinical neonatal aspects in view of congenital toxoplasmosis in cat and dog.

Chapter 8 - *Toxoplasma gondii* is an obligate intracellular parasite belonging to the phylum Apicomplexa, infecting all warm-blooded animals, with a worldwide distribution. Effective vaccines may contribute toward preventing and controlling the spread of toxoplasmosis. At present, only one commercial vaccine based on the live-attenuated S48 strain was developed for sheep and goats, while a vaccine for pigs, cats and humans is still lacking. Therefore, the focus of current review is to identify the protective antigens and develop antigen delivery systems. Searching the undiscovered vaccine candidates by genomics, transcriptomics, and proteomics is an effective approach.

On the other hand, many effective vaccine carriers have been investigated for their ability to induce a wide range of protective immune responses including humoral and cellular immunity, as well as protective effect.

This article presents the current status of vaccine strategies against toxoplasmosis, with a focus on the most advanced approaches using DNA-, virus- and protozoa-based vector vaccines.

Chapter 9 - Toxoplasmosis is a worldwide parasite disease caused by the aplicomplexa *Toxoplasma gondii.* This important parasitic infection remains persistently in infected individuals and may affect to both humans and animals. The diagnosis of toxoplasmosis has always been a challenge. Serology has been an usual tool for the detection of infection. However, given that toxoplasmosis is of great clinical relevance in pregnant women and immunosuppressed patients, there is always an increasing interest in developing alternatives for timely diagnosis to determine the presence and levels of parasitemia. The molecular diagnostic tools of *T. gondii* include the Polymerase Chain Reaction (PCR) with its variants, such as end-point PCR, real time PCR, and lamp, which permit a very specific determination of the genome of the protozoa from different biological samples. For this purpose PCR from amniotic fluid, placental and brain tissues, whole blood, cerebrospinal fluid, urine, vitreous fluid, aqueous humor, bronchoalveolar lavage fluid and pleural and peritoneal fluids has proved of value to diagnose *T.gondii.* The most common use of PCR is for prenatal diagnosis of the congenital infection using amniotic fluid samples. Several factor may influence the success of molecular detection of *T.gondii* such as the method of purification of DNA samples and very specific technical details that determine the sensitivity and specificity of diagnostic tests, such as the selection of primers, the use of hot start, the use of the enzyme uracyl-DNA-glycosylase to prevent carryover contamination, the size of the PCR product and use of internal control or nested PCR.

The aim of this chapter is to point out and discuss the current and more successful molecular biology techniques for the diagnosis and quantification of *Toxoplasma gondii* in clinical samples.

In: Recent Advances in Toxoplasmosis Research ISBN: 978-1-63117-914-3
Editor: Connor M. Lee

Chapter 1

FETAL AND MATERNAL TOXOPLASMOSIS

Helieh S. Oz**, DVM, Ph.D., AGAF
University of Kentucky Medical Center
Lexington, KY, US

ABSTRACT

Toxoplasmosis is one of the most important foodborne illness and fetal maternal inflammatory syndromes. Currently, there is no safe and effective approved therapy against fetal maternal complication or persistent chronic infection. *Toxoplasma* has a sexual stage in intestinal epithelia of the cats, to form resistant oocysts. A predominant source of human infection in North America is considered to be contaminated food and water with oocysts rather than cysts forms. Fetus becomes infected by transplacental transmission acquired from infected mom with an acute or the reactivation of the chronic or latent infection due to the stressors during pregnancy. *Toxoplasma* invades fetal central nervous system with adverse affect in brain neuro-structural development and pathological as well as psycho-behavioral alteration leading to mental retardation. T*oxoplasma* has a unique mind/brain altering effect with increased sexual attractions and is a sexually transmissible disease through contaminated semen. In this chapter, fetal maternal toxoplasmosis, complication, diagnosis, current therapies and a novel anti-fetal maternal toxoplasmosis therapy is discussed with a promising future for clinical trial.

* Email: Hoz2@email.uky.edu.

Keywords: Fetal Maternal, Congenital Toxoplasmosis, *Toxoplasma, Atovaquone*, Diclazuril

Background

Toxoplasma is an intracellular organism, and one of the most important sources of foodborne and congenital infection. About 1.5 billion people worldwide are predicted to have toxoplasmosis, frequently with unknown lifelong health consequences [1]. *Toxoplasma* is classified as "Category B pathogen" according the Center for Disease Control (CDC) and National Institute of Health (NIH), which once infect the host following acute stage; the organisms reside in muscles and brain in cyst forms for the lifetime and waiting for reactivation. *Toxoplasma* is an Apicomplexan protozoa with sexual stage which takes place in the intestinal epithelia of cats, where organisms replicate and mature to form resistant oocysts passed in the feces. Cats usually become infected first 6 months of their life and pass oocysts containing sporozoites for about 1-2 weeks. Humans and animals acquire systemic form of infection in asexual stage through consumption of contaminated animal products including milk, raw/undercooked meat and seafood or mature oocysts in water, fruits and vegetables.

Toxoplasma infects humans and animals, specifically in impoverish and socioeconomically disadvantage populations including women, African American, Hispanics, and Native Americans and is considered as a "common neglected disease of poverty" [2]. It is estimated that 1,500,000 cases of toxoplasmosis occurs in the United States each year and only 15% of these cases show clinical symptoms or are detected [3]. The pathogens which account for over 80% of food-related diseases and deaths are non-typhoid *Salmonella spp* (31%), *Listeria* (28%), and *Toxoplasma* (21%) [4]. According to a more recent study, the leading causes of foodborne hospitalization are non-typhoid *Salmonella spp* (35%), Norovirus (26%), *Campylobacter* (15%), and *Toxoplasma* (8%) while leading causes of death still remain *Salmonella* (28%) and *Toxoplasma* (24%) [5]. Therefore, *Toxoplasma* is considered as the 2nd [5] or 3rd major cause of foodborne death in the United States [4]. The *Toxoplasma* annual cost of illnesses is estimated $3 billion and the quality-adjusted life year loss is 11,000 QALYs in the United States [1].

Generally, *Toxoplasma* disseminates from the gut throughout the body, and the organisms seek refuge in the muscular tissues and central nervous system (CNS) in cyst forms during the dormant stage [6]. Extracellular tachyzoites readily infect the host cells including leucocytes, monocytes, macrophages and dendritics and exploit the host cells as "Trojan Horse" a) to disseminate throughout the body and to cross the blood brain barrier [7] as well as the placenta and b) to provide protection against host immune defense [8]. Toxoplasmosis in immunocompetent individuals is usually asymptomatic or manifested with general malaise as flu like syndrome and lymphadenitis, but outcomes can include severe pathological damages in immuneo-compromised patients as well as fetuses leading to demise and death [9].

Fetal Maternal Toxoplasmosis

Pregnant women infect their fetus when become acutely infected by ingesting oocysts contaminated food and water, or consuming cysts harboring bradyzoites-infected meat (Figure 1). Additionally, transplacental transmission is acquired by the reactivation of the chronic or latent infection due to the stressors including pregnancy and other immunosuppressors. In any circumstances, whether oocysts (sporozoites), or cysts (bradyzoites) are the origin of the infection the organisms transform to active infectious form of tachyzoites and propagate in the organs including uterus to cause the infection. Then the tachyzoites bypass the transplacental blood barrier to invade the fetus and to compromise the embryonic developmental process. A predominant source of human infection in North America is contaminated food and water with oocysts [10]. Of interest, sera and surveys were collected from 76 moms with congenital infected infants in 4 different epidemic areas and evaluated by the National Collaborative Chicago-based Congenital Toxoplasmosis Study (NCCCTS). The data revealed 78% of these moms had primary infection originated from oocysts while only 49% of these had direct contact with cats. Therefore, educational hygienic programs alone may benefit, but will not prevent severity of health and socioeconomic consequences associated with fetal maternal toxoplasmosis. Therefore, a possible effective cat vaccination program, implementation of systematic serological testing of pregnant women and newborns, followed by treatments may prevent fetal maternal toxoplasmosis in North America [10]. Brazil has a high rate of *Toxoplasma* infection as 50-80% of child-bearing women and 50% of children have antibodies titers. Also, 5 up to 23 of infants are found to be infected per 10,000 at birth in Brazil [11].

Congenital toxoplasmosis may manifest with a long list of complications including spontaneous miscarriage and abortion, fetal growth retardation, encephalomyelitis, intracranial calcifications, hydrocephalus, neurological, mental illnesses, retinochoroiditis, visual and auditory inflammatory disorders, cardiovascular abnormalities, and pains [12-16]. The severity of complications is dependent on the stage of gestation at which the fetus is infected, as the earlier the infection the more severe the consequences [12-13]. Those fetuses infected late in gestation may born normal, but develop symptoms of CNS and retinochoroiditis later in life and the new lesions may occur in untreated as well as treated children [12].

Other factors such as, genetic predisposition which affect immune response characteristics, including HLA may influence clinical outcomes [17-18]. As pregnancy progresses, maternal immune system faces a dual dilemma: to tolerate the growing semi-allogeneic fetus, at the same time to protect mom and offspring against pathogens. Indeed successful pregnancy requires an extremely delicate balance in regulation of the immune system at the materno-fetal interface resulting in tolerance (Th2) of the fetus [19-20]. The expression of the HLA-G molecules is responsible for reprogramming the local maternal immune response towards tolerance. The subsets of tolerogenic dendritic cells, DC-10 secrete high amounts of IL-10 and express high levels of HLA-G and its ligand ILT4 present in the peripheral blood which is essential to induce adaptive regulatory T cells. DC-10 and HLA-G-expressing $CD4^+$ T cells are highly present in human uterus decidual lining compared to peripheral blood in the first trimester of pregnancy, suggesting these may be accumulated or induced at the fetal maternal interface to promote tolerance [19].

Professional antigen presenting B cells in particular B-1a can activate or tolerize T cells, to participate either in generation or regulation of the immune response. B-1a B cells are involved in humoral immune response leading to pre-eclampsia, during pregnancy [21]. Similarly, in *Toxoplasma* infected mice, anti-mHSP70 autoantibody are released exclusively by CD5+ subset of B cells (B-1a cells) and not by conventional B cells (B-2 cells) [22]. The involvement of *Toxoplasma* infection in disorders is mainly associated with a strong Th1 infectious and immune-response that contributes to the pregnancy complications [23], possibly due to an altered balance and massive dysregulated immune response [24], rather than direct noxious affects of the pathogens. For instance, non-lethal infection with type II (ME49) *Toxoplasma* is characterized by a Th1 response elicit the release of IL-12 by macrophages, dendritic cells and neutrophils and the subsequent production of IFN-γ by NK cells and T cells. IFN-γ combined with TNFα, which induces formation of reactive oxygen and nitrogen intermediates, lead to nutrient deprivation, and control of parasite proliferation [25]. In contrast, IL-10 deficient mice produce higher levels of IFN-γ and IL-12 [26-27] which result in a fatal cytokine shock syndrome in infected mice [28]. Therefore, IL-10 likely plays an important role in modulating the levels of the immune response. In the brain, resident macrophages (MΦ, microglia) produce IFN-γ to recruit activated T cells to mediate immunity for controlling tachyzoites and the associated tissue damage [29]. In addition, microglia from infected animals tends to release nitric oxide (NO) to eliminate the organisms. The mechanisms by which microglia activities contribute to destructive or protective functions in the CNS remain to be determined.

Toxoplasmosis Reactivation

Toxoplasmosis reactivation occurs primarily during pregnancy, in AIDS and in immunocompromised individuals including bone marrow and organ transplantation when cysts wall rupture and organisms are released to access blood and lymphatic cells to spread the infection. Congenital toxoplasmosis in humans as well as animals (e.g. sheep, goats, dogs) is initiated by the transplacental transmission of organisms during maternal infection [30]. Congenital toxoplasmosis caused by a reactivation, or as an acquired infection during pregnancy is known to be associated with an altered equilibrium of immune response and inflammation led by pathogens [30-32]. Fetal maternal toxoplasmosis results in an extensive immune and inflammatory response to the organisms in the gastrointestinal tissues with a low number of pathogenic burdens as demonstrated in a pregnancy model [33]. Indeed, managing the inflammation is vital in order to prevent damage to the host and the nested fetus during the infection. In fact, surge of uncontrolled inflammatory response in toxoplasmosis can be fatal during the pathogenic clearance [33].

The congenital transmission of toxoplasmosis was first reported in a 3 day old infant from New York in 1939 [31], and the importance of maternal fetal transmission has long been recognized for several decades [32]. Massachusetts Department of Health estimated that one case of congenital toxoplasmosis occurs for every 10,000 births. Therefore, from 4,000,000 live births in the United States, about 400 children are estimated to have congenital toxoplasmosis [4]. Fetal maternal toxoplasmosis leads to spontaneous abortion, intrauterine fetal death or severe congenital defects, such as encephalitis, hydrocephaly and chorioretinitis [34]. A retrospective trail was performed on 12035 pregnant women in the period of 2000-2011 in Buenos Aires, Argentina. The prevalence rate of anti-*Toxoplasma* antibody was 18.33% (2206/12035), and 37 out of 9792 susceptible women were presented with acute infection and incidence rate of 3.8 per 1000 births with transplacental transmission rate of 5.4% [35].

FETAL MATERNAL TOXOPLASMOSIS AND MENTAL DISORDERS

Toxoplasma invades the central nervous system with adverse affect in brain neuro-structural development and pathological as well as psycho-behavioral alteration leading to mental retardation [36-38]. More recently, maternal exposure or latent *Toxoplasma* infection has been linked to a potential increased risk for autism and schizophrenic episodes and this hypothesis has received a considerable scientific and media attention. In addition, Over 40 studies have confirmed an increased prevalence of toxoplasmosis among schizophrenic patients [39].

Toxoplasma infection may evolve brain dopamine alterations [40-41]. According a longitudinal study, women with chronic toxoplasmosis had a higher risk of self-harm and accidents [42]. Another cross-sectional study indicated that *Toxoplasma* seropositive individuals demonstrate increased risk of nonfatal suicidal aggression [43]·

Pregnant women with latent toxoplasmosis have higher proportion of infants with genetic or developmental disorders in offspring. These include premature fetuses in about 16th week of gestation, with slower rates of development in the first trimester as well as postnatal motor development in infants of moms with latent toxoplasmosis. For instance, these infants have significant delayed in the ability to control their heads (p=0.039), due to decreased strength of embryonic quality control related to immunosuppression caused by infection in mothers. As some of these defects are related to diarrheal malnutrition or severe acute illness contributed to severity of congenital toxoplasmosis, cognitive and developmental deficits [44].

In a 20 year 3 large retrospective and one case control prospective trials on military personnel, university students, pregnant women and blood donors have shown that even the asymptomatic *Toxoplasma* infection greatly influences various aspects of human life [39]. The infected subjects differed from uninfected controls in the personality profiles suggesting that

Toxoplasma influences personality rather than personality influences the probability of infection. These changes were elevated reaction time causing increased probability of traffic accidents in infected subjects. Latent toxoplasmosis was associated with immunosuppression, and extremely high prevalence of infected mothers to have children with Down syndrome. *Toxoplasma*-infected male students appeared to be more masculine with dominant personality and involved in the initiation of severe forms of schizophrenia than those uninfected students [39].

Another trail evaluated 190 school children in rural area for seropositive and seronegative, developmental age, body mass, height, physical fitness, grades and the risk factors of infection as the presence of cats in the household and eating raw meat products. The prevalence of anti-*Toxoplasma* antibodies was 41% amongst children and the rate of infection higher in girls (44%) than in boys (36%) as measured by IFAT and ELISA tests. The developmental age measured with electrophoretical mobility of nuclei was significantly higher while school performance significantly lower for *Toxoplasma* infected girls compared to uninfected matched controls. As expected those boys who ate raw meat products were most likely to be seropositive [45]. In addition, a recent surveillance obtained between 2000-2012 in Nepal, reported congenital toxoplasmosis as second (to malaria) highest annual parasitic burden with 9255 Disability-Adjusted Life Year (95%) and Credibility Interval of 6135-13,292 [46].

FETAL MATERNAL TOXOPLASMOSIS AND CRANIOFACIAL MALFORMATION

It is estimated that 1/3 of all babies born with birth defects, display some sort of anomalies of the head and face. These include cleft lip, cleft palate, small or absent facial and skull bones, malformed, eyes, and teeth [47]. Craniofacial disorders are a primary cause of infant mortality and have serious lifetime consequences [47]. The Center for Disease Control estimates the lifetime cost of treating children born each year with cleft lip, cleft palate alone to be $697 million. In addition, oral and craniofacial disorders are the main cause of non-dental orofacial pain but the etiology and pathophysiology poorly understood. Approximately 10–15% of adults have persistent and recurrent orofacial pain [48-50] that impact their daily life. Of these, 50% to 70% report myofascial as the principal source of their pain [48-50]. Thus far, the relationship between congenital toxoplasmosis and incidence of craniofacial disorders has not been understood. Although, *Toxoplasma* cysts and associated inflammations has been reported in the craniofacial region, including tongues, salivary ducts, tonsils, buccal tissues, cleft lips and palates from infected neonates [51-57]. Mothers and neonates with orofacial clefts have significantly higher titers for *Toxoplasma* and inflammatory cytokines in their saliva compared to normals [51-52]. In addition, toxoplasmosis can cause skeletal muscle disorders, with severe neuropathic and inflammatory pain and increased myogenic serum enzymes [58-59]. This indicates that toxoplasmosis may be a possible cause of oral and craniofacial disorders in addition to other complications such as Cleft palate, skeletal muscle deformation, salivary gland inflammation, tonsillitis, and cervical lymphadenopathy. These limited reports are consistent with fetal maternal toxoplasmosis being a possible risk factor for oral and craniofacial disorders.

Organ Transplantation Blood Transfusion

Organ transplant patients including liver, lung, bone marrow, pancreas and kidney recipients are at risk for toxoplasmosis as a result of immunosuppressive therapy and contaminated organ or reactivation of chronic infection followed by high mortality rate if not detected. Toxoplasmosis is referred as an underestimated complication following hematopoietic stem cell transplantation and blood transfusion [60]. It is usually detected in autopsy or remains undetected due to the non-specific symptoms and lack of clinical awareness of healthcare individuals [61]. Toxoplasmosis may manifest with clinical symptoms of acute or recurrent abdominal pain and pancreatitis [62-63]. Chronic progressive pancreatitis may be associated with fat necrosis, inflammation, obstruction of bile duct, focal hepatic necrosis, elevated amylase and lipase serum values, and abdominal fat with yellowish plaques formation. Pancreas becomes firm in palpation and white in color, with adhesions and gall bladder distended with pale color bile. The bile duct forms tortuous and dilated and small hepatic bile ducts prominent. *Toxoplasma* organisms can be detected in the pancreatic tissue, acinar cells and bile duct epithelium [64- 65]. In Japan while, the incidence rate of toxoplasmosis in transplant patients is low (1.8%) but the mortality in these infected patients is reported to be very high [60]. Toxoplasmosis is frequently difficult to detect and potentially fatal in kidney transplant recipients. As an example, a patient who received *Toxoplasma* positive kidney allograft developed invasive toxoplasmosis 10 days after surgery, with symptoms of high fever, skin rash, arthralgia, and renal failure, followed by anemia, thrombocytopenia, liver dysfunction, pneumonia, and encephalitis. No organism was detected in blood smears, alveolar fluid, renal graft biopsy, with negative brain computed tomography. However, patient passed with septic shock on day 11 when organisms were detectable in bone marrow aspirate [66].

Women with renal disease become pregnant and pregnancy is generally very high risk in those with chronic renal insufficiency, end-stage renal disease, dialysis patients and transplant recipients. Hypertension is the most common life-threatening problem in these moms. Transplant recipients are at risk for infections that can infect the fetus, including *Toxoplasma.* Renal disease patients have an increased risk for prematurity and intrauterine growth restriction. For women who conceive after starting dialysis, the probability of a surviving infant is reduced to 50% [67-68]. Therefore, pregnant transplant recipients need to be monitored for *Toxoplasma* as well as other opportunistic infections [68].

Allogeneic bone marrow and peripheral blood stem cell transplantation are recommended treatment for some malignant hematologic diseases, such as marrow failure syndromes, and severe congenital immunodeficiency conditions [69]. Fetal thrombocytopenia can be caused by maternal immunological complications as well as infectious diseases including toxoplasmosis [70]. In a retrospective study of over 5000 fetal blood samples 7% had thrombocytopenia due to congenital infectious disease (*Toxoplasma, Rubella* and *Cytomegalovirus*) of which 26% had toxoplasmosis [70]. Indeed, thrombocytopenia is more common during congenital toxoplasmosis than purpura [71]. While, unusual cases of maternal and neonatal toxoplasmosis may occur during late third trimester and infants develop severe unexplained systemic disease including disseminated intravascular coagulopathy with thrombocytopenia, hepatitis, jaundice and pneumonitis [72].

TOXOPLASMOSIS AND AUTOIMMUNE DISEASE

Toxoplasma is implicated in several autoimmune disorders. While, etiological factors in the induction of autoimmune disease remain elusive, a possible link with toxoplasmosis may exist. Immunosuppressants, and monoclonal antibodies such as anti-TNF which are widely used in healthcare for the treatment of autoimmune diseases and organ transplantation may result in acute toxoplasmosis in these patients. However, the interaction and mechanism between the development of acute toxoplasmosis and immunosuppressant therapy are not fully understood. Sera of 1514 patients with 11 different autoimmune diseases from health centers in Europe and Latin America as well as 437 control samples from geographically matched areas studied for the prevalence of anti-*Toxoplasma* antibodies IgG and IgM and serum autoantibodies [73]. Anti-*Toxoplasma* antibody IgG was positive in 42% of patients versus 29% of controls ($p<0.0001$). Anti-*Toxoplasma* antibody IgG was associated with anti-phospholipid syndrome ($p<0.0001$), ANCA-associated vasculitides ($p<0.01$), autoimmune thyroid diseases ($p<0.0001$), systemic sclerosis ($p<0.0001$), rheumatoid arthritis ($p<0.0001$) and cryoglobulinemia ($p<0.0001$). Anti- *Toxoplasma* antibody IgM was more prevalent in patients with anti-phospholipid syndrome ($p<0.01$), systemic sclerosis ($p<0.05$) and inflammatory bowel disease ($p<0.05$) than in controls. These findings support the notion that *Toxoplasma* contributes to the pathogenesis of autoimmune disease [73]. Chronic inflammatory bowel disease (IBD) mainly Crohn's disease and ulcerative colitis is regarded as autoimmune response to gut microbiota, and toxins from gram negative lipopolysaccharid (LPS), bypassing the compromised epithelium by underlying dysregulated oral tolerance [74-75]. In addition, the use of immunosuppressives in IBD patients may increase the risk of opportunistic diseases and *Toxoplasma* infection. The greatest risks of infections may relate to the combined use of immunomodulating agents rather than to individual drugs [76]. Those IBD patients treated with corticosteroids, azathioprine, methotrexate, cyclosporine, and TNF-blocking biological are more susceptible to infections than others. Crohn's patients are prone for gut abscess formation followed by infectious complications as well as toxoplasmosis. This alerts the physicians treating patients with IBD to be aware of the risk for infectious as well as of strategies to minimize these infectious complications in these patients [76].

Peroral *Toxoplasma* infection provokes small intestine necrosis and death and in many ways mimics IBD. Macrophage migration inhibitory factor is important for controlling parasite burden and survival against *Toxoplasma* infection by increasing local as well as systemic inflammation, which results in tissue damage and death in macrophage migration inhibitory factor (MIF) deficient mice. Lack of MIF suppressed pro-inflammatory responses at the ileal mucosa and reduced TNFα, IL-12, IFN-γ and IL-23 cytokines levels, while increased expression of IL-22 in ileal mucosa. MIF also affected the expression of matrix metalloproteinase-9 (MMP-9) in the intestine of infected mice. Systemic inflammatory cytokines in the plasma and liver damage were less in MIF deficient mice compared to wild-type animals, suggesting MIF may controls *Toxoplasma* infection while increasing local and systemic inflammation, tissue damage and death [77].

Severe colonic inflammatory response is observed in pregnancy model for toxoplamosis, associated with significant shortening in colonic length, with infiltration of lymphocytes, and macrophages and microabscess formations in the cryptic structures in infected dams [33,78-79].

IBD models for ulcerative colitis often utilize chemical induction for inflammation in the gut to evaluate the mechanisms of disease progression. Oral administration of dextran sulfate sodium (DSS) for 3-16 cycles [74] induces chronic inflammation with elevated gram negative gut microbiota. Pathogen-associated molecular patterns (PAMPs) derived from intestinal microbial which may modulate IBD by the interaction with innate immune receptors, are Toll-like receptors (TLRs) and macrophage patent recognition associated receptors [80-81]. Colitis significantly increases colonic lipopeptide (4-fold) and LPS equivalent to 550-fold in concentrations. Similarly, *Toxoplasma* induced ileitis drastically increases ileal concentrations of lipopeptide (370-fold), and LPS (3,300-fold) $P<0.01$. Therefore, induction of colitis or ileitis is associated with significant disease-specific alterations to the PAMP profile of the gut microbiota and *Toxoplasma* infection [80]. Sera from 119 patients with IBD and 98 healthy controls were assessed for anti-*Toxoplasma* antibody. Titer of anti-*Toxoplasma* was higher in IBD patients than controls suggesting that *Toxoplasma* is involved in the pathogenesis of IBD, and especially in Crohn's disease in patients [82].

Toxoplasmosis may be associated with anorexia or obesity by altering inflammatory fat distribution as organisms alter and reside in fatty tissues [83]. However, no association is reported between anti-*Toxoplasma* IgG antibody and obesity in 985 individuals from Iceland, Sweden and Estonia [84]. In contrast, excessive gestation weight gain is reported in pregnant women with toxoplasmosis compared with uninfected pregnant women [85,39] as well as in a pregnancy model that mimics human toxoplasmosis complications [33,78-79]. Similarly *Toxoplasma* infection is reported to cause increased weight gain and atrophy of myenteric neurons of the jejunum in animals [86].

Lipoprotein lipase which regulates plasma triglyceride clearance and distribution among tissues is predominately involved in infection-induced hypertriglyceridemia, by modulating adipose and muscle lipoprotein lipase activity in toxoplasmosis [87]. *Toxoplasma* may alter weight gain by reducing muscle lipoprotein lipase and modulating tissue lipoprotein lipase activity during chronic infection to promote triglyceride distribution in adipose tissue

[87]. In addition, *Toxoplasma* lacks ability to synthesize sterol for growth and replication and scavenging on the host blood cholesterol through the low density lipoprotein receptors. Yet, *Toxoplasma* infection causes an exaggerated Th1 systemic inflammatory response which enhances pro-atherogenic effects [88-89]. Finally, while inflammation is crucial for the host defense and survival against pathogens, non-resolving chronic and excessive inflammatory response damages tissues as implicated in *Toxoplasma* infection involvement in these autoimmune disorders [83].

Toxoplasma and Sexual Attraction

Recent studies reveal that *Toxoplasma* has a mind/brain altering effect with increased sexual attractions as infected rats seek cat's urine odor, while uninfected rats' response with rapid innate defensive behaviors and fear to avoid cats [90-91]. This is to fulfill the *Toxoplasma* requirement for the sexual propagation in final host, cats by consumption of the infected and brain impaired rats and small rodents. Indeed *Toxoplasma* infection alters neural activity in limbic brain areas necessary for innate defensive behavior and increases activity in adjacent limbic regions of sexual attraction when infected rat is exposed to cat urine odor [90]. Furthermore, toxoplasmosis is a sexually transmissible disease as organisms are transmitted by contaminated semen. Artificial vaginal insemination with tachyzoites contaminated semen can infect goats with 80% embryonic resorption (4/5) [92] and in dogs [93] as well as vertical transmission in infected ewes during natural mating with infected sheep [94]. There is a potential transmission route in *Toxoplasma* infected semen during artificial insemination (inoculation) or natural mating. These studies demonstrate possible sexual transmission of *Toxoplasma* with consequent vertical transmission to their offspring.

Fetal Maternal Toxoplasmosis Diagnostics

Toxoplasma infection during pregnancy is a serious health risk factor for the fetus. Thus, quick and accurate diagnostics are essential for possible preventions and available therapeutics. Fetal maternal toxoplasmosis is commonly diagnosed using serological assays to detect types and levels of anti-*Toxoplasma* antibodies. Blood test is required to be repeated during the pregnancy and also suggested at the time of birth. As the importance of congenital toxoplasmosis is well known, pregnant women are routinely tested in Austria, France, Italy, Portugal, and Uruguay for antibodies detections. In addition, limited screening program are used in Germany, Switzerland and Belgium. Pre- and neonatal screening for congenital toxoplasmosis are performed on more than two million pregnant women every year in Europe, North and South America at the estimated cost of more than 500 million dollars annually [95]. However, United States does not require routine screening of pregnant women for toxoplasmosis. Considering significant variation of the disease manifestation and cosmopolitan distribution of *Toxoplasma* infection, it is recommended that infants with severe unexplained systemic disease to be tested for possible congenital toxoplasmosis [72]. Seronegative pregnant women indicating no previous exposure to infection are at risk for the infection and recommended to be serology tested monthly until birth.

Standard laboratory diagnosis of toxoplasmosis is based on the presence of IgM and IgG anti-*Toxoplasma* antibodies, and molecular technology used as alternative tools to increase sensitivity [96]. Typically, infection is associated with high levels of anti-*Toxoplasma* IgM antibody followed by a rise in IgG levels 1 to 3 weeks after infection. However, atypical infection with IgG sero-conversion happens in pregnancy without detectable IgM levels. These cases are very difficult to diagnose in congenital toxoplasmosis [97]. Those pregnant women with low and steady levels of IgG anti-*Toxoplasma* antibody have been previously exposed to the organism and fetus may remain safe. However, detection of IgM or elevation of IgG anti-*Toxoplasma* antibodies suggest a new acquired or reactivation of chronic/latent infection due to possible immunosuppression with a threat of infection to the fetus. Therefore, amniotic fluid exam can be performed to determine health status of the fetus and possible exposure to the infection.

Sabin-Feldman dye test is a complement-lysis-based assay with relative sensitivity and specificity to measure anti-*Toxoplasma* IgG antibodies and the international "gold standard" for diagnosis of toxoplasmosis. The Sabin-Feldman dye test is considered to be somehow more reliable than commercially available ELISA kits in some labs, but the test is time consuming and requires live organisms treated with each serum dilution to be analyzed under the microscope [98].

In serious cases of neurological disorders including visual and auditory impairments, IgM and IgG antibodies combined with cerebrospinal fluid (CSF) polymerase chain reaction (PCR) is recommended to detect *Toxoplasma*

DNA. From 58 infants (0 to 180 days) born of the infected moms, CSF PCR was positive in 46.5% and 100% negative in uninfected healthy infants. PCR was positive in 80% of those infants with hydrocephalus, 53% in cerebral calcifications and 60% of those with eye complications. Therefore, infants with neurological disorders, IgM and IgA antibodies combined with CSF PCR, are considered to yield a higher sensitivity for diagnosis of congenital toxoplasmosis when compared with each test alone [99].

In addition, the new multiplex, BioPlex® 2200 automated analyzer (Bio-Rad Laboratories, Hercules, CA) and ToRC IgG/IgM kit can detect anti-*Toxoplasma* antibodies in the same assay and is considered superior to Platelia IgG/IgM ELISA test (Bio-Rad Laboratories) or Toxo-Screen Direct Agglutination assay (bioMérieux, Lyon, France) with 91.3% specific and 97.8% sensitive to detect IgG and IgM, thus yielding more precise diagnosis of acute *Toxoplasma* infection [100].

Other serological tests to detect specific IgG and IgM in blood samples are the indirect fluorescent antibody test (IFAT), microparticle enzyme immunoassay (MEIA) and enzyme-linked fluorescent assay (ELFA) used according the manufacturer's instructions. The IgM sensitivity is reported 60% and specificity 100% except for IFAT with 92% and for ELISA-IgA of 57% respectively [101].

The molecular techniques include Western Blot analysis to detect anti-*Toxoplasma* IgM and IgA in infected infants [102]. The real-time PCR assay has been shown to be the best-performing technique to detect DNA in amniotic fluid with 98% sensitivity and 100% specificity compared to other conventional PCR and nested PCR, or multiplex-nested-PCR techniques similarly utilizing B1 gene primers [96].

α-Fetoprotein analysis, is a biomarker for fetal development and birth defects. α-fetoprotein (AFP) is useful in the prediction of fetal placental development and growth. Elevations of maternal AFP have been associated with pregnancy, liver diseases, tumors, fetal death and resorption [103]. Serum AFP binds and transport bilirubin, steroids, and drugs. AFP has been recognized as both a B- and T-cell regulatory protein [104]. Elevated levels of AFP are also indicators for fetal distress conditions like fetal maternal transfusion, pre-eclampsia, fetal retardation and demise. Maternal serum AFP assay may be useful in predicting immune responses and intrauterine death in maternal toxoplasmosis [105].

Common *Toxoplasma* staining Procedures: Bradyzoites in cysts and free tachyzoites in infected tissue biopsies are detected using immunohistochemical staining, Giemsa and other direct staining methodologies.

Immunohistochemical staining (IHC): The paraffin-embedded sections are cut, deparaffinized with xylene, rehydrated in alcohol baths, washed in PBS with 0.1% bovine serum albumin (BSA), then quenched for endogenous peroxidase activity by incubating in 3% hydrogen peroxide in methanol 30 min, and blocked with rabbit serum (Dako #N1699) for 30 min. The sections are incubated with poly or monoclonal anti-*Toxoplasma* antibody, diluted 1:500 for 90 min and developed with DAB-Chromogen (DakoCarpenteria, CA) for about 5 min until signal developed and subsequently counterstained with hematoxylin then ammonia treated, dehydrated stepwise through alcohol, and cleared in xylene [33].

Giemsa staining: Giemsa is a delicate polychromatic stain that reveals a fine nuclear detail of *Toxoplasma* organisms. Giemsa stain contains Methylene Blue Azure Basic dyes combined with Eosin Acidic dyes. The deparaffinized slide sections are stained with the polychromatic Giemsa (40 drops/50 ml distilled water) to stain nuclei of the *Toxoplasma* organisms and to permit differentiation among the cells. Then, the slides are depreciated in 1% Glacial acetic acid, dehydrated in alcohol and xylene series and mounted in synthetic resin on slides [33].

Fetal and Maternal Toxoplasmosis and Therapeutic Approaches

Thus far, there is no safe and effective or FDA approved therapy against fetal maternal toxoplasmosis or any drug treatment capable of eliminating the persistent and chronic infection [106]. Present therapies for toxoplasmosis are pyrimethamine, sulfasalazine, sulfadiazine and spiramycin alone or associated with pyrimethamine plus sulfadoxine used to prevent transfer of *Toxoplasma* from the actively infected mother to the fetus. Postpartum treatment of fetal and maternal toxoplasmosis with sulfadiazine and pyrimethamine has remained almost unchanged for over 5 decades. Recently, sulfadoxine, has replaced sulfadiazine with a longer half-life to provide basis for a dose schedule with higher compliance [95]. However, this approach is not always effective and associated with potential adverse effect and treatment with these potentially fetotoxic drugs must be considered [106-110]. In fact, pyrimethamine is a pregnancy category C drug and can cause severe side effects such as bone marrow suppression in both infant as well as mother. In addition, spiramycin a macrolide antibiotic is used for a few decades in

Europe, Latin America and Canada but is considered as an experimental therapy in United States. Spiramycin monotherapy is effective only when administered in early pregnancy principally as preventive measure and not after fetus exposed to the organisms. More than ½ of patients who receive spiramycin may retain *Toxoplasma* DNA in their peripheral blood as they continue to remain infected [109]. In a prospective cohort performed in 246 newborns in risk for congenital toxoplasmosis in Brazil (2003- 2011), 58% of infants from treated moms were born with congenital toxoplasmosis of which 18.6% had severe infection. In contrast 115 untreated moms gave birth to 73% of newborns with congenital infection of which 60.7% had severe infection [101]. In a 20 year prospective clinical trial (1985-2005) of infected mothers (666) treated with spiramycin, alone or combined with pyrimethamine plus sulfadoxine with live born children, 112 (17%) newborns were confirmed with congenital toxoplasmosis, and 26% later developed chorioretinitis [111]. Similarly, in another study in France, from 257 live birth from women with prenatal positive diagnosis treated with both spiramycin and pyrimethamine plus sulfadoxine, 66 (24%) children were diagnosed infected with the transmission rates of toxoplasmosis 7% in the first, 24% second, and 59% in third trimesters, respectively [112]. While, spiramycin is known as a fairly safe drug with minor gastrointestinal side effects, a case report indicates of significant fetal bradycardia with the use of spiramycin [110]. Other fetal maternal treatments are azithromycin, clarithromycin, atovaquone, dapsone, and cotrimoxazole (trimethoprim-sulfamethoxazole), however, their efficacy have not been proven. The available studies are either observational investigations of referred patients or observational studies accrued over many years, often decades. [95].

Given these circumstances, there is a great need for more effective therapeutic modalities with less toxicity and better tolerated regiments for fetal and congenital toxoplasmosis as well as for the recurrent *Toxoplasma* related disease.

Atovaquone

Current therapy against toxoplasmosis includes atovaquone (hydroxy-1,4-naphthoquinone) which is an FDA approved treatment but not for the use in fetal maternal toxoplasmosis and small children [106]. Recent experimental studies demonstrate atovaquone to protect the fetuses and the dams from the infection as well as *Toxoplasma* induced mild to moderate inflammatory complications. Atovaquone has been proven to be effective against tachyzoites and cyst forms of *Toxoplasma* and malarial infections [113], opportunistic *Pneumocystis* pneumonia [114], and blood borne *Babesia microti* causative of human babesiosis and endemic in North Eastern, and New England area [115-116].

Atovaquone impairs fungal and parasite respiration by binding to the ubiquinol oxidation site of cytochrome bc1 complex [117] and selectively targets the mitochondrial function to collapse their membrane [118]. The radiolabelled tracing studies have shown that atovaquone mainly attaches to the plasma protein (99%) with a half life of 1.5 to 3 days and 2 peaks; the 1st peak appears at 1h-8h and 2nd in 1-4 days after a single oral dose used in volunteers. Surgical biliary tubes installed in patients demonstrate that atovaquone is exclusively (94%) excreted from the body through the feces and it is not metabolized [119]. As mice with a targeted gene mutation in the interferon regulatory factor 8 when latently infected with *Toxoplasma*, develop reactivated encephalitis, and those treated with atovaquone are protected against encephalitis and death [120]. Furthermore, atovaquone treatment is advantageous over the standard therapy with pyrimethamine plus sulfadiazine or combination of pyrimethamine plus clindamycin based on the inflammatory responses in the brain parenchyma, and the number of the organisms located in the brain of mice [120]. In addition, atovaquone is detectable in sera, brains, livers, and lungs from infected mice utilizing high pressure liquid chromatography (HPLC) and Mass Spectroscopy [120]. Atovaquone overall is not associated with severe adverse reactions in the recommended dosages and has a reasonably favorable profile with no lymphocytes cytotoxic effects [121]. Atovaquone was shown to have limited but significant protective effects against gastrointestinal complications in animals. Dams showed significant excess weight gain ($p<0.001$) due to the inflammatory response to the *Toxoplasma* infection [33]. The excess weight gain in infected animals are in accord with a retrospective cohort trial in 194 infected pregnant women who gained more weight compared to 785 uninfected moms ($P <0.001$) [122]. However, atovaquone had minor effect on the excess body weight gain in dams [33].

Overall, atovaquone was shown to be fairly safe and to protect against inflammatory aspects of the fetal maternal progression of toxoplasmosis.

Diclazuril and Fetal Maternal Toxoplasmosis

Diclazuril [4-chlorophenyl [2,6-dichloro-4-(4,5-dihydro-3H-3,5-dioxo-1,2,4-triazin-2-yl)pheny l acetonitrile] is related to herbicides and currently used in poultry and livestock industry to protect against coccidian diseases.

As a member of the phylum Apicomplexan, *Toxoplasma* contains a highly conserved region of non-photosynthetic protochlorophyllidae with traces of rudimentary plant chloroplast epitope and not present in mammals. Apicoplast is an extranuclear DNA organelle, visible in tachyzoites under light microscopy, and has an extensnive similarity to the plant vacuoles, to carry transcriptional and translational device in *Toxoplasma* with specific enzymes unwinding DNA. Apicoplast is possibly acquired by secondary endosymbiosis relationship originated between eukaryotic *Ciliate* ancestor and prokaryotic green alga in evolution [123]. Therefore, apicoplast has a unique sensitivity to herbicide related compounds which make it safe and attractive region in infected humans and animals as a desirable drug discovery and vaccine target against *Toxoplasma* with a metabolic pathway absent in the human and animals.

Diclazuril and its related benzeneacetonitriles substances specifically target the chloroplast derived chlorophyll a-D1 complex [124]. Therefore, diclazuril binds the chloroplast epitope and interacts with the D1 protein of the *Toxoplasma* apicoplast without damaging the mammalian host cells. In addition, diclazuril is shown to downregulate expression of serine/threonine protein phosphatase in second-generation merozoite of *Eimeria tenella* to induce apoptosis [125]. Serine/threonine protein phosphatase has about 98% homology in *Toxoplasma* that demonstrates a possible mechanism of action for diclazuril.

Diclazuril is shown to be a safe compound [126] with no recognized drug side effects as used at therapeutic dose levels. Diclazuril is rapidly absorbed following oral administration to achieve steady-state concentration in plasma and cerebrospinal fluid [78]. Therefore, diclazuril has potential with anti-*Toxoplasma* therapeutic efficacy and minimal mammalian toxicity. Our recent studies have shown diclazuril to be safe in pregnancy in general and effective in fetal maternal toxoplasmosis [78-79]. While atovaquone protects against some aspects of gastrointestinal complications in experimental congenital toxoplasmosis in murine [33], diclazuril has a superior efficacy against anemia, colonic length improvement, hepatic complications and excess body weight as consequence of toxoplasmosis [78]. This novel compound warrants future clinical trials in fetal maternal and chronic toxoplasmosis.

Murine Models for Fetal Maternal Toxoplasmosis

Murine play an important role in propagation and transmission of *Toxoplasma* and are commonly used in studying toxoplasmosis, as they mimic well the human infection. The majority of *Toxoplasma* strains isolated from North America and Europe belong to three clonal lineages I, II and III, of which types I and II are associated with congenital toxoplasmosis [127]. The congenital toxoplasmosis models are induced by the oral inoculation of *Toxoplasma* cysts, tachyzoites from infected animals [128], or intraperitoneal injection of cysts from ME49 strain [129]. Studies indicates that a dose of 10,000 bradyzoites or 100 oocysts of the *Prugniaud* strain (Type II) to cause 50% congenital infection of the rat litters. In contrast, lactation alone does not support transmission of infection from dams to the neonates [128]. CD1 mice are hardy animals with relatively large number of pups and routinely used in pregnancy investigations [33,78,81]. Recently, a relatively simple and reliable murine model was induced to mimic *Toxoplasma* reactivation or contaminated blood transfusion and organ transplantation, by evading oral inoculation to instigate congenital toxoplasmosis. The fetal maternal model relies on a moderate to severe systemic infectious and inflammatory syndrome for the use in drug discovery and evaluation [33]. In this model, fetal health is compromised by the invasion of pathogens encountered with inflammatory responses from infected dam through the mechanism of transplacental transmission and in a dose related manner [33]. This model shorten the induction of infection period and bypasses 1) *in vivo* serial passage of the organisms and the use of surrogate mice to propagate the organisms and 2) the requirement for oral tract inoculation of a large number of organisms by using direct intraperitoneal inoculation of tachyzoites obtained from *in vitro* cell cultures. The model mimics the process of the intrauterine infection to study progression of toxoplasmosis in fetal maternal complications. In addition, this model eliminated the use of surrogate cats to develop oocysts and possible environmental contamination with persistent oocysts. For this model, genotype II tachyzoites (ME-49) was used to initiate the infection in the model as is most frequently associated with the human disease and congenital toxoplasmosis in North America [127].

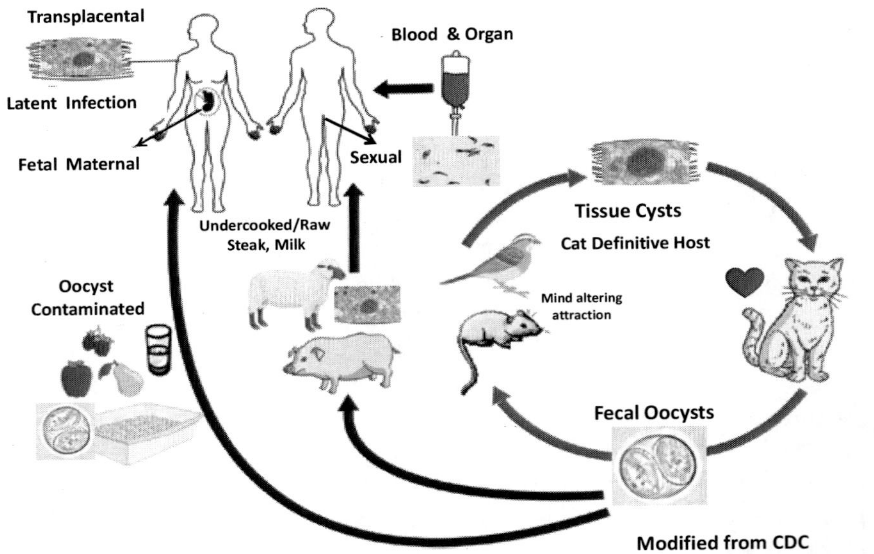

Figure 1. Routes of Transmission.

CONCLUSION

Toxoplasmosis is one of the most important foodborne illness and fetal maternal inflammatory syndromes. Over a century after discovery, currently there is no safe and effective treatment against chronic and persistent infection or fetal maternal toxoplasmosis. Toxoplasmosis commonly remains under or undetected due to the non-specific symptoms and lack of clinical awareness of healthcare individuals. A predominant source of infection is contaminated food and water with oocysts rather than cysts forms. Fetus becomes infected by transplacental transmission acquired from infected mom with an active infection due to the stressors during pregnancy. *Toxoplasma* invades fetal central nervous system with adverse affect in brain neuro-structural development as well as psycho-behavioral alteration leading to mental retardation. T*oxoplasma* has a unique mind/brain altering effect with increased sexual attractions and is a sexually transmissible disease through infected semen. Given these circumstances, there is a great need for more effective therapeutic modalities with less toxicity and better tolerated regiments for fetal and congenital toxoplasmosis as well as for the recurrent *Toxoplasma* related disease. Promising novel anti-*Toxoplasma* agents include diclazuril and its related compounds targeting rudimentary plant chloroplast epitope not present in man warrant future clinical trials.

Funding Support: This work was supported in part by a grant from National Institutes of Health NIH-DE019177 (H. Oz).

REFERENCES

[1] Hoffmann S, Batz MB, Morris JG Jr. Annual cost of illness and quality-adjusted life year losses in the United States due to 14 foodborne pathogens. *J. Food Prot.* 2012 Jul;75(7):1292-302. doi: 10.4315/0362-028X.JFP-11-417.

[2] Hotez PJ. Neglected Infections of Poverty in the United States of America. *PLOs ONE* 2008, 2:256:1-11.

[3] Jones JL, Kruszon-Moran D, Wilson M, Mcquillan G, Navin T, Mcauley JB. *Toxoplasma gondii* infection in the United States: Seroprevalence and risk factors. *Amer. J.Epidemiol.* 2001;154:357–365.

[4] Mead PS, Slutsker L, Dietz V, McCaig LF, Bresee JS, Shapiro C, Griffin PM, Tauxe R V. Food-related illness and death in the United States. *Emerg. Infect. Dis.* 1999,5: 606–625.

[5] Scallan E, Hoekstra RM, Angulo FJ, Tauxe RV, Widdowson M-A, Roy SL, Jones JL, Griffin PM. Foodborne Illness Acquired in the United States Major Pathogens. *Emerg. Infect. Dis.* www.cdc.gov/eid • Vol. 17, No. 1, January 2011

[6] Prandota J. The importance of *Toxoplasma gondii* infection in diseases presenting with headaches. Headaches and aseptic meningitis may be manifestations of the Jarisch-Herxheimer reaction. *Int. J.Neurosci.* 2009;119(12):2144-82. Review.

[7] Bierly AL, Shufesky WJ, Sukhumavasi W, Morelli AE, Denkers EY. Dendritic Cells Expressing Plasmacytoid Marker PDCA-1 Are Trojan Horses during *Toxoplasma gondii* Infection. *J.Immunol.* 2008,18: 8485–8491.

[8] Elsheikha HM, Khan NA. Protozoa traversal of the blood brain barrier to invade the central nervous system. *FEMS Microbiol. Rev.* 2010, 34 532–553.

[9] Dubey JP, Jones JL. *Toxoplasma gondii* infection in humans and animals in the United States. *Int. J.Parasitol.* 2008;38:1257-78.

[10] Boyer K, Hill D, Mui E, Wroblewski K, Karrison T, Dubey JP, Sautter M, Noble AG, Withers S, Swisher C, Heydemann P, Hosten T, Babiarz J, Lee D, Meier P, McLeod R. Toxoplasmosis Study Group. Unrecognized ingestion of *Toxoplasma gondii* oocysts leads to congenital toxoplasmosis and causes epidemics in North America. *Clin. Infect. Dis.* 2011 Dec;53(11):1081-9. doi: 10.1093/cid/cir667.

[11] Dubey JP, Lago EG, Gennari SM, Su C, Jones JL. Toxoplasmosis in humans and animals in Brazil: high prevalence, high burden of disease, and epidemiology. *Parasitology* 2012 Sep;139(11):1375-424. doi: 10.1017/S0031182012000765.

[12] Dunn D, Wallon M, Peyron F, Petersen E, Peckham C, Gilbert R. Mother-to child transmission of toxoplasmosis: Risk estimates for clinical counseling. *Lancet* 1999, 353,1829–1833

[13] Remington JS, McLeod R, Thulliez P, Desmonts G. Toxoplasmosis. In ''Infectious Diseases of the Fetus and Newborn Infant'' (Remington JS, Klein JO, Wilson CB, Baker CJ, eds), 6th edn, 2006, pp. 947–1091. Philadelphia: Elsevier Saunders.

[14] Gilbert R, Gras L. Effect of timing and type of treatment on the risk of mother to child transmission of *Toxoplasma gondii*. *Bjog*2003:110: 112–120.

[15] Gras L, Wallon M, Pollak A, Cortina-Borja M, Evengard B, et al. Association between prenatal treatment and clinical manifestations of congenital toxoplasmosis in infancy: a cohort study in 13 European centres. *Acta.Paediatr.*2005:94: 1721–1731.

[16] McLeod R, Boyer K, Karrison T, Kasza K, Swisher C, et al. Outcome of treatment for congenital toxoplasmosis, 1981–2004: the National Collaborative Chicago-Based, Congenital Toxoplasmosis Study. *Clin. Infect. Dis.*2006: 42: 1383–1394.

[17] Mack DG, Johnson JJ, Roberts F, Roberts CW, Estes RG, et al. HLA class II genes modify outcome of *Toxoplasma gondii* infection. *Int. J.Parasitol.*1999:29:1351–1358.

[18] Jamieson SE, de Roubaix L-A, Cortina-Borja M, Tan HK, Mui EJ, et al. Genetic and epigenetic factors at COL2A1 and ABCA4 Influence clinical outcome in congenital toxoplasmosis. *PLoS ONE* 2008, 3: e2285. doi:10.1371/journal.pone.0002285.

[19] Muzzio DO, Soldati R, Rolle L, Zygmunt M, Zenclussen AC, Jensen F. B-1a B Cells Regulate T Cell Differentiation Associated with Pregnancy Disturbances. *Front Immunol.* 2014; 5: 6. 2014 January 21. doi: 10.3389/fimmu.2014.00006.

[20] Norwitz ER, Schust DJ, Fisher SJ. Implantation and the survival of early pregnancy. *N. Engl. J. Med.*2001, 345, 1400–1408.

[21] Amodio G1, Mugione A, Sanchez AM, Viganò P, Candiani M, Somigliana E, Roncarolo MG, Panina-Bordignon P, Gregori S. HLA-G expressing DC-10 and CD4(+) T cells accumulate in human decidua during pregnancy. *Hum.Immunol.* 2013 Apr;74(4):406-11. doi: 10.1016/j.humimm.2012.11.031.

[22] Chen M1, Aosai F, Mun HS, Norose K, Hata H, Yano A. Anti-HSP70 autoantibody formation by B-1 cells in *Toxoplasma gondii*-infected mice. *Infect.Immun.* 2000 Sep;68(9):4893-9.

[23] Romero R, Espinoza J, Mazor M. Can endometrial infection/inflammation explain implantation failure, spontaneous abortion, and preterm birth after in vitro fertilization? *Fertil.Steril* 2004, 82, 799–804.

[24] Senegas A, Villard O, Neuville A, Marcellin L, Pfaff AW, Steinmetz T, Mousli M, Klein JP, Candolfi E, *Toxoplasma gondii*-induced foetal resorption in mice involves interferon-cinduced apoptosis and spiral artery dilation at the maternofoetal interface. *Int J Parasitol* 2009,39: 481–487.

[25] Sibley LD, Mordue DG, Su C, Robben PM, Howe DK. Genetic approaches to studying virulence and pathogenesis in *Toxoplasma gondii. Philos Trans. R. Soc.Lond B. Biol. Sci.* 2002, 29;357:81-8.

[26] Oz HS, Chen T, de Villiers WJS. Green Tea Polyphenols and Sulfasalazine have Parallel Anti-inflammatory Properties in Colitis Models, *Front Immunol 2013,* 4, 132:1-10.

[27] Oz HS, Ray M, Chen T, McClain C. Efficacy of a TGF-β2 Containing Nutritional Support Formula in a Murine Model of IBD. *J. Amer Coll Nutri* 2004, 23: 220-226.

[28] Gazzinelli RT, Wysocka M, Hieny S, Scharton-Kersten T, Cheever A, Kühn R, Müller W, Trinchieri G, Sher A. In the absence of endogenous IL-10, mice acutely infected with *Toxoplasma gondii* succumb to a lethal immune response dependent on CD4+ T cells and accompanied by overproduction of IL-12, IFN-gamma and TNF-alpha. *J.Immunol.* 1996 Jul 15;157(2):798-805.

[29] Rozenfeld C, Martinez R, Figueiredo RT, Bozza MT, et al. Soluble factors released by *Toxoplasma gondii*-infected astrocytes down-modulate nitric oxide production by gamma interferon-activated microglia and prevent neuronal degeneration. *Infect. Immun.* 2003;71:2047-57.

[30] Buxton D, Thomson K, Maley S, Wright S, Bos HJ. Vaccination of sheep with a live incomplete strain (S48) of *Toxoplasma gondii* and their immunity to challenge when pregnant. *Vet. Rec.* 1991;129:89–93.

[31] Wolf A, Cowen D, Paige B. Human toxoplasmosis: occurrence in infants as an encephalomyelitis verification by transmission to animals. *Science* 1939, 89, 226–227.

[32] Jones JL, Lopez A, Wilson M, Schulkin J, Gibbs R. Congenital toxoplasmosis: A review. *Obst. Gynecol.Surv.* 2001,56: 296–305.

[33] Oz HS, Tobin T. Atovaquone Ameliorates Gastrointestinal Toxoplasmosis Complications in a Pregnancy model. *Med. Sci. Mon.* 18, 2012, pp. BR337-345.

[34] Wong SY, Remington JS. Toxoplasmosis in pregnancy. *Clin. Infect. Dis.* 1994, 18:853–861.

[35] Carral L, Kaufer F, Olejnik P, Freuler C, Durlach R. [Prevention of congenital toxoplasmosis in a Buenos Aires hospital]. *Medicina* (B Aires). 2013;73(3):238-42.

[36] Brown AS, Schaefer CA, Quesenberry CP Jr, Liu L, Babulas VP, Susser ES. Maternal exposure to toxoplasmosis and risk of schizophrenia in adult offspring.*Am. J. Psychiatry* 2005;162:767-73.

[37] Bachmann S, Schröder J, Bottmer C, Torrey EF, Yolken RH. Psychopathology in first-episode schizophrenia and antibodies to *Toxoplasma*gondii. *Psychopathology* 2005;38:87-90.

[38] Wang HL, Wang GH, Li QY, Shu C, Jiang MS, Guo Y. Prevalence of *Toxoplasma* infection in first-episode schizophrenia and comparison between *Toxoplasma*-seropositive and *Toxoplasma*-seronegative schizophrenia.*ActaPsychiatr. Scand.*2006;114:40-8.

[39] Flegr J. Influence of latent *Toxoplasma* infection on human personality, physiology and morphology: pros and cons of the *Toxoplasma*-human model in studying the manipulation hypothesis.*J. Exp. Biol.*2013 Jan 1;216(Pt 1):127-33. doi: 10.1242/jeb.073635.

[40] Fekadu A, Shibre T, Cleare AJ. Toxoplasmosis as a cause for behaviour disorders--overview of evidence and mechanisms. *Folia. Parasitol* 2010 Jun;57(2):105-113.

[41] Torrey EF, Bartko JJ, Lun ZR, Yolken RH. Antibodies to *Toxoplasma gondii* in patients with schizophrenia: a meta-analysis. *Schizophr. Bull* 2007 May;33(3):729-736.

[42] Pedersen MG, Mortensen PB, Norgaard-Pedersen B, Postolache TT. *Toxoplasma gondii* infection and self-directed violence in mothers. *Arch Gen Psych* 2012 Nov;69(11):1123-1130.

[43] Zhang Y, Traskman-Bendz L, Janelidze S, et al. *Toxoplasma gondii* immunoglobulin G antibodies and nonfatal suicidal self-directed violence. *J clin psychiatry* 2012 Aug;73(8):1069-1076.

[44] Kaňková S, Sulc J, Křivohlavá R, Kuběna A, Flegr J. Slower postnatal motor development in infants of mothers with latent toxoplasmosis during the first 18 months of life. *Early Hum. Dev.* 2012 Nov;88(11):879-84. doi: 10.1016/j.earlhumdev.2012.07.001.

[45] Mizgajska-Wiktor H, Jarosz W, Andrzejewska I, Krzykała M, Janowski J, Kozłowska M. Differences in some developmental features between *Toxoplasma gondii*-seropositive and seronegative school children. *Folia Parasitol* (Praha). 2013 Nov;60(5):416-24.

[46] Devleesschauwer B, Ale A, Torgerson P, Praet N, Maertens de Noordhout C, Pandey BD, Pun SB, Lake R, Vercruysse J, Joshi DD, Havelaar AH, Duchateau L, Dorny P, Speybroeck N. The burden of parasitic zoonoses in Nepal: a systematic review. *PLoSNegl. Trop. Dis.* 2014 Jan 2;8(1):e2634. doi: 10.1371/journal.pntd.0002634. eCollection 2014.

[47] Trainor PA. Craniofacial birth defects: The role of neural crest cells in the etiology andpathogenesis of Treacher Collins syndrome and the potential for prevention. Stowers Institute for Medical Research, Kansas City, Missouri. *Am. J. Med. Genet. A.* 2010 Dec;152A(12):2984-94. doi: 10.1002/ajmg.a.33454. Review.

[48] Drangsholt MT, LeResche L, Ramsey DS, Herring S, Dworkin SF. Comments on pediatric internal derangements. *Am. J.Orthod.Dentofacial. Orthop.* 1994 Mar;105(3):38A-39A.

[49] Dunn KM, Jordan KP, Mancl L, Drangsholt MT, Le Resche L. Trajectories of pain inadolescents: a prospective cohort study. *Pain* 2011 Jan;152(1):66-73.

[50] Macfarlane TV, Kenealy P, Kingdon HA, Mohlin B, Pilley JR, Mwangi CW, Hunter L, Richmond S, Shaw WC. Orofacial pain in young adults and associated childhood andadulthood factors: results of the population study, Wales, United Kingdom. *Community Dent Oral Epidemiol.* 2009 Oct;37(5):438-50.

[51] Holková R, Molnárová A, Nemec R, Brozman M, Fábry J, Horáková E. [Relation between toxoplasmosis and orofacial clefts in children]. *Bratisl Lek Listy.* 1994,95:64-7.

[52] Gu SZ, Lu S, Ma YW. [Study on the relationship between congenital toxoplasmosis andmonsters of cleft lip and palate accompanied by multiple malformation]. *Shanghai KouQiang Yi Xue.* 1992;1:66-9.

[53] Gabka J. [Etiology of cleft palate, with special reference to toxoplasmosis.] *Dtsch Zahnarztl* Z. 1954 Sep 15;9:1043-7.

[54] Gabka J. [Etiology of labial, oral and palatal fissures with special reference toToxoplasmosis.] *Dtsch Stomatol*. 1953 ;3:294-300.

[55] Glass RB, Fernbach SK, Norton KI, Choi PS, Naidich TP. The Infant Skull: A Vault of Information. *Radiographics* 2004; 24:507–522.

[56] Amendoeira MR, Coutinho SG. Isolation of *Toxoplasma gondii* from the saliva and tonsils ofa three-year-old child. *J. Infect. Dis*. 1982;145:587.

[57] Köybaşi S, Süslü AE, Yigit B, Boran C. Acquired toxoplasmosis of the buccal area with extranodular involvement: report of an unusual case. *Ear Nose Throat J*. 2009;88:E12-4.

[58] Calore EE, Minkovski R, Khoury Z, Seguro AC, Perez Calore NM, Cavaliere MJ. Skeletalmuscle pathology in 2 siblings infected with *Toxoplasma gondii*. *J.Rheumatol*. 2000; 27:1556-9.

[59] Pergola G, Cascone A, Russo M. Acute pericarditis and myocarditis by *Toxoplasma gondii* in an immunocompetent young man: a case report. *Infez Med*. 2010;18:48-52.

[60] Sumi M, Aosai F, Norose K, Takeda W, Kirihara T, Sato K, Fujikawa Y, Shimizu I, Ueki T, Hirosima Y, Ueno M, Ichikawa N, Watanabe M, Kobayashi H. Acute exacerbation of *Toxoplasma gondii* infection after hematopoietic stem cell transplantation: five case reports among 279 recipients. *Int. J.Hematol*. 2013 Aug;98(2):214-22. doi: 10.1007/s12185-013-1379-8. Epub 2013 Jun 8.

[61] Munir A, Zaman M, Eltorky M. *Toxoplasma gondii* pneumonia in a pancreas transplant patient. *South Med. J*. 2000 Jun;93(6):614-7.

[62] Dudley NJ, Balfour AH. Non-Hodgkin's lymphoma presenting as 'chronic activetoxoplasmosis' *Postgrad Med. J,* 1988 Nov;64(757):883-885.

[63] Parenti DM, Steinberg W, Kang P. Infectious causes of acute pancreatitis. *Pancreas* 1996 Nov;13(4):356-71.

[64] Smart ME, Downey RS, Stockdale PH. Toxoplasmosis in a cat associated with cholangitis and progressive pancreatitis. *Can. Vet. J*. 1973 Dec;14(12):313-6.

[65] Petrak M, carpenter J. Feline toxoplasmosis. *J. Am. Vet. Med. Ass*. 1965; 146: 728-734.

[66] Segall L, Moal MC, Doucet L, Kergoat N, Bourbigot B. Toxoplasmosis-associated hemophagocytic syndrome in renal transplantation. *Transpl Int*. 2006 Jan;19(1):78-80.

[67] Hou S. Pregnancy in chronic renal insufficiency and end-stage renal disease. *Am. J. Kidney Dis.* 1999 Feb;33(2):235-52.

[68] Hou S. Pregnancy in renal transplant recipients. *Adv. Ren. Replace Ther.* 2003 Jan;10(1):40-7.

[69] Ordemann R, Petzold K, Hölig K, Schaffer B, Mauersberger S, Ehninger G. Experiences of the Dresdner Cord Blood Bank, supported by the Deutsche Knochenmarkspenderdatei. *Semin.Thromb.Hemost.* 1999;25(6):575-8.

[70] Hohlfeld P, Forestier F, Kaplan C, Tissot JD, Daffos F. Fetal thrombocytopenia: a retrospective survey of 5,194 fetal blood samplings. *Blood.* 1994 Sep 15;84(6):1851-6.

[71] Michez D, Quintart C, Noël E, Lepage P. [Peripheral thrombopenicpurpura associated with acquired toxoplasmosis]. *Rev. Med.Brux.* 1998 Jun;19(3):135-7.

[72] Armstrong L, Isaacs D, Evans N. Severe neonatal toxoplasmosis after third trimester maternal infection. *Pediatr Infect. Dis. J.* 2004 Oct;23(10):968-9. *Pediatr Infect. Dis. J.* 2004 Oct;23(10):968-9.

[73] Shapira Y, Agmon-Levin N, Selmi C, Petríková J, Barzilai O, Ram M, Bizzaro N, Valentini G, Matucci-Cerinic M, Anaya JM, Katz BS, Shoenfeld Y. Prevalence of anti-Toxoplasma antibodies in patients with autoimmune diseases. *J.Autoimmun.* 2012 Aug;39(1-2):112-6. doi: 10.1016/j.jaut.2012.01.001.

[74] Oz HS, Chen T, Ebersole JL, A Model for Chronic Mucosal Inflammation in IBD and *Periodontitis Dig. Dis. Sci.* DOI 10.1007/s10620-009-1031-x

[75] Brandtzaeg P. Inflammatory bowel disease: Clinics and pathology. Do inflammatory bowel disease and periodontal disease have similar immunopathogeneses? *Acta Odontol. Scand.* 2001;59: 235–243.

[76] Epple HJ. Therapy- and non-therapy-dependent infectious complications in inflammatory bowel disease. *Dig. Dis.* 2009;27(4):555-9. doi: 10.1159/000233297.

[77] Cavalcanti MG, Mesquita JS, Madi K, Feijó DF, Assunção-Miranda I, Souza HS, Bozza MT. MIF participates in *Toxoplasma gondii*-induced pathology following oral infection. *PLoS One.* 2011;6(9):e25259. doi: 10.1371/journal.pone.0025259.

[78] Oz HS, Tobin T. Diclazuril protects against maternal gastrointestinal syndrome and congenital toxoplasmosis. *Int. J.Clin. Med.*, Special issue: Treatment of liver diseases, 2014, 5, 93-101, Online January 2014 (http://www.scirp.org/journal/ijcm)

[79] Oz HS, de Villiers WJ. Novel synergistic protective efficacy of Atovaquone and Diclazuril on fetal-maternal toxoplasmosis. *Mediator Inflamm* 2014 (in press)

[80] Erridge C, Duncan SH, Bereswill S, Heimesaat MM. The induction of colitis and ileitis in mice is associated with marked increases in intestinal concentrations of stimulants of TLRs 2, 4, and 5. *PLoS One.* 2010 Feb 9;5(2):e9125. doi: 10.1371/journal.pone.0009125.

[81] Oz HS, Ebersole J, de Villiers W. The Macrophage Pattern Recognition Scavenger Receptors SR-A and CD36 protect against microbial induced pregnancy loss. *Inflam Res.* 2011:60:93–97.

[82] Lidar M, Langevitz P, Barzilai O, Ram M, Porat-Katz BS, Bizzaro N, Tonutti E, Maieron R, Chowers Y, Bar-Meir S, Shoenfeld Y. Infectious serologies and autoantibodies in inflammatory bowel disease: insinuations at a true pathogenic role. *Ann. N Y Acad. Sci.* 2009 Sep;1173:640-8. doi: 10.1111/j.1749-6632.2009.04673.x.

[83] Carter CJ. Toxoplasmosis and Polygenic Disease Susceptibility Genes: Extensive *Toxoplasma gondii* Host/Pathogen Interactome Enrichment in Nine Psychiatric or Neurological Disorders. *CarterJ.Pathog.* 2013;2013:965046. doi: 10.1155/2013/965046.

[84] Thjodleifsson B, Olafsson I, Gislason D, Gislason T, Jögi R, Janson C. Infections and obesity: A multinational epidemiological study. *Scand. J. Infect. Dis.* 2008;40(5):381-6.

[85] Kaňková S, Sulc J, Flegr J. Increased pregnancy weight gain in women with latent toxoplasmosis and RhD-positivity protection against this effect. *Parasitology.* 2010 Oct;137(12):1773-9. doi: 10.1017/S0031182010000661.

[86] Hermes-Uliana C, Pereira-Severi LS, Luerdes RB, Franco CL, da Silva AV, Araújo EJ, Sant'AnaDde M. Chronic infection with *Toxoplasma gondii* causes myenteric neuroplasticity of the jejunum in rats. *Auton Neurosci.* 2011 Feb 24;160(1-2):3-8. doi: 10.1016/j.autneu.2010.09.003.

[87] Picard F, Arsenijevic D, Richard D, DeshaiesY. Responses of adipose and muscle lipoprotein lipase to chronic infection and subsequent acute lipopolysaccharide challenge. *Clin.Diagn Lab.Immunol.* 2002 Jul;9(4):771-6.

[88] Portugal LR, Fernandes LR, Alvarez-Leite JI. Host cholesterol and inflammation as common key regulators of toxoplasmosis and artherosclerosis development. *Expert Rev. Anti. Infect.Ther.* 2009;7(7):807-19. doi: 10.1586/eri.09.60.

[89] Lige B, Sampels V, Coppens I. Characterization of a second sterol-esterifying enzyme in *Toxoplasma* highlights the importance of cholesterol storage pathways for the parasite. *Mol.Microbiol.* 2013;87(5):951-67. doi: 10.1111/mmi.12142.

[90] House PK, Vyas A, Sapolsky R. Predator cat odors activate sexual arousal pathways in brains of *Toxoplasma gondii* infected rats. *PLoS One*. 2011;6(8):e23277. doi: 10.1371/journal.pone.0023277.

[91] Knight K. How pernicious parasites turn victims into zombies. *J. Exp. Biol.* 2013 Jan 1;216(Pt 1):i-iv.

[92] Wanderley FS, Porto WJ, Câmara DR, da Cruz NL, Feitosa BC, Freire RL, de Moraes EP, Mota RA. Experimental vaginal infection of goats with semen contaminated with the "CPG" strain of *Toxoplasma gondii*. *J.Parasitol.* 2013 Aug;99(4):610-3. doi: 10.1645/12-126.1.

[93] Arantes TP, Lopes WD, Ferreira RM, Pieroni JS, Pinto VM, Sakamoto CA, Costa AJ. *Toxoplasma gondii*: Evidence for the transmission by semen in dogs. *Exp.Parasitol.* 2009 Oct;123(2):190-4. doi: 10.1016/j.exppara.2009.07.003.

[94] Lopes WD, Rodriguez JD, Souza FA, dos Santos TR, dos Santos RS, Rosanese WM, Lopes WR, Sakamoto CA, da Costa AJ. Sexual transmission of *Toxoplasma gondii* in sheep. *Vet.Parasitol.* 2013 Jul 1;195(1-2):47-56. doi: 10.1016/j.vetpar.2012.12.056.

[95] Petersen E, Schmidt DR. Sulfadiazine and pyrimethamine in the postnatal treatment of congenital toxoplasmosis: what are the options? *Expert Rev.Anti InfectTher.* 2003;1:175-82.

[96] Teixeira LE, Kanunfre KA, Shimokawa PT, Targa LS, Rodrigues JC, Domingues W, Yamamoto L, Okay TS. The performance of four molecular methods for the laboratory diagnosis of congenital toxoplasmosis in amniotic fluid samples. *Rev. Soc. Bras Med. Trop.* 2013 Sep-Oct;46(5):584-8.

[97] Fricker-Hidalgo H, Cimon B, Chemla C, Darde ML, Delhaes L, L'ollivier C, Godineau N, Houze S, Paris L, Quinio D, Robert-Gangneux F, Villard O, Villena I, Candolfi E, Pelloux H. *Toxoplasma* seroconversion with negative or transient immunoglobulin M in pregnant women: myth or reality? A French multicenter retrospective study. *J.Clin.Microbiol.* 2013 Jul;51(7):2103-11. doi: 10.1128/JCM.00169-13.

[98] Dando C, Gabriel KE, Remington JS, Parmley SF. Simple and efficient method for measuring anti-*Toxoplasma* immunoglobulin antibodies in

human sera using complement-mediated lysis of transgenic tachyzoites expressing beta-galactosidase. *J.Clin.Microbiol.* 2001 Jun;39(6):2122-5.

[99] Olariu TR, Remington JS, Montoya JG. Polymerase Chain Reaction in Cerebrospinal Fluid for the Diagnosis of Congenital Toxoplasmosis. *Pediatr. Infect. Dis. J.* 2014 Jan 17..

[100] Guigue N, Menotti J, Hamane S, Derouin F, Garin YJ. Performance of the BioPlex(R) 2200 flow immunoassay (Bio-Rad) in critical cases of serodiagnosis of toxoplasmosis. *Clin. Vaccine Immunol.* 2014 Jan 29. [Epub ahead of print].

[101] Avelino MM, Amaral WN, Rodrigues IM, Rassi AR, Gomes MB, Costa TL, Castro AM. Congenital toxoplasmosis and prenatal care state programs. *BMC Infect. Dis.* 2014 Jan 18;14:33. doi: 10.1186/1471-2334-14-33.

[102] di Carlo P, Romano A, Casuccio A, Cillino S, Schimmenti MG, Mancuso G, la Chiusa S, Novara V, Ingrassia D, Li Vecchi V, Trizzino M, Titone L. Investigation and management of *Toxoplasma gondii* infection in pregnancy and infancy: a prospective study. *Acta Pharmacol. Sin.* 2011 Aug;32(8):1063-70. doi: 10.1038/aps.2011.55.

[103] Mizejewski GJ. Physiology of Alpha-Fetoprotein as a Biomarker for Perinatal Distress: Relevance to Adverse Pregnancy Outcome. *Exp. Biol.Med.* 2007, 232:993–1004.

[104] Ritter M, Ali MY, Grimm CF, Weth R, Mohr L, Bocher WO, Endrulat K, Wedemeyer H, Blum HE, Geissler M. Immunoregulation of dendritic and T cells by alpha-fetoprotein in patients with hepatocellular carcinoma. *J.Hepatol.* 2004, 41:999-1007.

[105] Kaur M, Verma IC. Serum alpha feto-protein screening in high risk pregnancies. *Indian J.Pediatr.* 1995;62:101-7.

[106] Cortina-Borja M, Tan HK, Wallon M, Paul M, Prusa A, Buffolano W, Malm G, Salt A, Freeman K, Petersen E, Gilbert RE. European Multicentre Study on Congenital Toxoplasmosis (EMSCOT). Prenatal treatment for serious neurological squeal of congenital toxoplasmosis: an observational prospective cohort study. *PLoS Med.* 2010,12;7. pii: e1000351.

[107] Daffos F, Forestier F, Capella-Pavlovsky M, Thulliez P, Aufrant C, Valenti D et al. Prenatal management of 746 pregnancies at risk for congenital Toxoplasmosis. *N. Engl. J. Med.* 1998;318:271-275.

[108] Berrebi A, Assouline C, Bessieres MH, Lathiere M, Cassaing S, Minville V, Ayoubi JM. Long-term outcome of children with congenital toxoplasmosis. *Am. J. Obstet. Gynecol.* 2010;203:552.e1-6.

[109] Habib FA. Post-treatment assessment of acute *Toxoplasma* infection during pregnancy. *J. Obstet.Gynaecol.* 2008;28:593-5.

[110] Julliac B, Theophile H, Begorre M, Richez B, Haramburu F. Side effects of spiramycin masquerading as local anesthetic toxicity during labor epidural analgesia. *Int. J. Obstet.Anesth* 2010;19:331-2.

[111] Berrébi A, Assouline C, Bessières MH, Lathière M, Cassaing S, Minville V, Ayoubi JM. Long-term outcome of children with congenital toxoplasmosis. *Am. J. Obstet. Gynecol.* 2010 Dec;203(6):552.e1-6. doi: 10.1016/j.ajog.2010.06.002.

[112] Bessières MH, Berrebi A, Cassaing S, Fillaux J, Cambus JP, Berry A, Assouline C, Ayoubi JM, Magnaval JF. Diagnosis of congenital toxoplasmosis: prenatal andneonatal evaluation of methods used in Toulouse University Hospital andincidence of congenital toxoplasmosis. *Mem. Inst. Oswaldo Cruz* 2009;104:389-92.

[113] Hudson AT, Dickins M, Ginger CD, Gutteridge WE, Holdich T, Hutchinson DB, Pudney M, Randall AW, Latter VS. 566C80: a potent broad spectrum anti-infective agent with activity against malaria and opportunistic infections in AIDS patients. *Drugs Exp.Clin. Res.* 1991;17:427-35.

[114] Oz HS, Hughes W, Rehg J. A rat model for dual opportunistic pathogens: *Cryptosporidium parvum* and *Pneumocystis carinii. Lab. Animal Sci.* 1999;49:331-334.

[115] Hughes W, Oz HS. Successful prevention and treatment of babesiosis with atovaquone. *J. Infect. Dis.* 1995;172:1042-1046.

[116] Oz HS, Westlund KH. "Human Babesiosis" an emerging transfusion dilemma. *Int. J.Hepatol.* 2012, Volume 2012, Article ID 431761, 5 pages doi:10.1155/2012/431761.

[117] Freyre A, Falcon J, Mendez J, Gonzalez M. *Toxoplasma gondii*: an improved rat model of congenital infection. *Exp.Parasitol.* 2008;120:142-6.

[118] Srivastava IK, Vaidya AB. A mechanism for the synergistic antimalarial action of atovaquone and proguanil. *Antimicrob. Agents Chemother* 1999;43:1334-9.

[119] Rolan PE, Mercer AJ, Tate E, Benjamin I, Posner J. Disposition of atovaquone in humans. *Antimicrob. Agents Chemother* 1997;41:1319-21.

[120] Dunay IR, Heimesaat MM, Bushrab FN, Muller RH, Stocker H, Arasteh K, Kurowski M, Fitzner R, Borner K, Liesenfeld O. Atovaquone Maintenance Therapy Prevents Reactivation of Toxoplasmic

Encephalitis in a Murine Model of Reactivated toxoplasmosis. *Antimicrob. Agents Chempther* 2004, 48, 4848–4854.

[121] Dinter D, Gajski G, Garaj-Vrhovac V. An alkaline comet assay study on the antimalarial drug atovaquone in human peripheral blood lymphocytes: a study based on clinically relevant concentrations. *J Appl Toxicol* 2013, 33,56-62. doi: 10.1002/jat.1711.

[122] Kaňková S, Sulc J, Flegr J. Increased pregnancy weight gain in women with latent toxoplasmosis and RhD-positivity protection against this effect. *Parasitology.* 2010 Oct;137(12):1773-9. doi: 10.1017/S0031182010000661.

[123] Köhler S, Delwiche CF, Denny PW, Tilney LG, Webster P, Wilson R J M., Jeffrey D. Palmer, David S. Roos. A Plastid of Probable Green Algal Origin in Apicomplexan Parasites *Science* 1997: 275, 1485 – 1489. DOI: 10.1126/science.275.5305.1485.

[124] Hackstein JH, Mackenstedt U, Mehlhorn H, Meijerink JP, Schubert H, Leunissen JA. Parasitic apicomplexans harbor a chlorophyll a-D1 complex, the potential target fortherapeutic triazines. *Parasitol. Res.*1995;81:207-16.

[125] Zhou W, Quan JH, Lee YH, Shin DW, Cha GH. *Toxoplasma gondii* Proliferation Require Down-Regulation of Host Nox4 Expression via Activation of PI3 Kinase/Akt Signaling Pathway. *PLoS One.* 2013 Jun 18;8(6):e66306. Print 2013.

[126] Assis RC, Luns FD, Beletti ME, Assis RL, Nasser NM, Faria ES, Cury MC. Histomorphometry and macroscopic intestinal lesions in broilers infected with *Eimeria acervulina. Vet.Parasitol.* 2010 Mar 25;168(3-4):185-9. doi: 10.1016/j.vetpar.2009.11.017. Epub 2009 Dec 16.

[127] Ajzenberg D, Cogne N, Paris L, Bessieres MH, Thulliez P, Filisetti P, Pelloux H, Marty P, Darde ML. Genotype of 86 *Toxoplasma gondii* isolates associated with human congenital Toxoplasmosis, and correlation with clinical findings. *J. Infect. Dis.*2002;186:684–689.

[128] Dubey JP, Ferreira LR, Martins J, McLeod R. Oral oocyst-induced mouse model of toxoplasmosis: effect of infection with *Toxoplasma gondii* strains of different genotypes, dose, and mouse strains (transgenic, out-bred, in-bred) on pathogenesis and mortality. *Parasitology* 2011,14:1-13.

[129] Takahashi J, Fukuda T, Tanaka J, Minamitani M, Onouchic K, Makiokad A. Bax-induced apoptosis not demonstrated in the congenital toxoplasmosis in mice. *Brain Dev* 2001, 23: 50±53.

[130] Araujo FG, Slifer T. Different Strains of *Toxoplasma gondii* Induce Different Cytokine Responses in CBA/Ca Mice. *Infect. Immun.* 2003, 71:4171-414.

In: Recent Advances in Toxoplasmosis Research ISBN: 978-1-63117-914-3
Editor: Connor M. Lee

Chapter 2

TOXOPLASMA GONDII, SUICIDE AND HOMICIDE

David Lester
The Richard Stockton College of
New Jersey, Galloway, NJ, US

ABSTRACT

Studies of European nations have found that the prevalence of the brain parasite *Toxoplasma gondii* is positively associated with both suicide and homicide rates. In addition, research on individuals has shown that the presence of *T. gondii* is associated with fatal and non-fatal suicidal behavior in both men and women. The mediating physiological processes for these associations may involve the neurotransmitter dopamine, the amino acid tryptophan and the hormone testosterone, all of which are impacted by the presence of *T. gondii.*

INTRODUCTION

Lafferty (2006) reported that the prevalence of a common brain parasite (*Toxoplasma gondii*) in 31 nations was associated with national measures of neuroticism. Since regional levels of neuroticism have been found to be associated with regional suicide rates (Voracek, 2009),[1] Lester (2010a) explored whether the national prevalence of this brain parasite was associated with national suicide rates. He obtained data for 20 European nations and found that the Pearson correlation between the prevalence of *T. gondii* in nations and male suicide rates was 0.55 and for female suicide rates 0.48. Lester introduced controls for the gross domestic product per capita, and these correlations were not greatly impacted (partial correlations of 0.44 and 0.46, respectively).

Lester (2010b) next compared the power of the prevalence of *T. gondii* versus other indices in predicting European suicide rates. In previous research, Lester (1987; Kondrichin and Lester, 1997) found that the percentage of Finno-Ugrians[2] in European countries and the proportion with type O blood also predicted European suicide rates. For 17 European nations with available data, all three indices were significant associated with suicide rates: the prevalence of *T. gondii* 0.55, the percentage of Finno-Ugrians 0.56 and the proportion with type O blood -0.55 for male suicide rates, and 0.48, 0.48, and -0.47, respectively for female suicide rates. In a multiple regression, only the prevalence of *T. gondii* and the proportion of Finno-Ugrians contributed significantly to the prediction of suicide rates.

A study by Ling et al. (2011) qualified this finding. By looking at suicide rates by age and sex, Ling et al. found that the association was significant only for women over the age of 45, and they noted that the prevalence of *T. gondii* in European countries is based primarily on blood tests on pregnant women, which might explain the narrowness of this association. Lester (2012) explored whether the same association could be found for homicide rates in the same sample of 20 European nations and found an association of 0.43, but for this association, introducing a control for the gross domestic product per capita reduced the size of the association to 0.22.[3]

---

[1] Voracek (2009) found this association over the American states but not over nations of the world (Voracek, 2006).

[2] An ethnic group that includes many Hungarians and Finns.

[3] The association between the gross domestic product per capita and the prevalence of *T. gondii* was -0.52, indicating that the incidence was greater in the poorer European nations in the sample.

RESEARCH IN INDIVIDUALS

Are these associations also found in studies of individuals? Five studies have been published.

Arling, et al. (2009) studied 218 patients diagnosed with an affective disorder (major depression or bipolar disorder) of whom 89 had made a prior suicide attempt. Blood samples were drawn from each patient and tested for the antibodies to *T. gondii*. Suicidal patients with recurrent depression had higher mean levels of antibodies than nonsuicidal patients with recurrent depression or normal controls.[4] The number of attempts and the psychiatric diagnosis were not associated with the level of antibodies.

Yagmur, et al. (2010) compared 200 attempted suicides in Turkey with 200 normal controls and found that significantly more of the attempted suicides were seropositive for *T. gondii* than the normal controls (41% versus 28%).

Okusaga, et al. (2011) tried to replicate this result in 950 schizophrenic patients, 351 of whom had a made a prior suicide attempt. The presence of antibodies was significant for those patients under the age of 38, but not for older patients. For the younger patients, the unadjusted odds ratio for suicide attempt history was 1.66 (95% confidence interval 1.12 to 2.46).[5] In this study, Okusaga, et al. also measured antibodies to cytomegalovirus, herpes simplex virus type 1 and gliadin, but these levels were not associated with a history of attempted suicide.

Pedersen, et al. (2012) followed a cohort of 45,788 women for 11-14 years who had tested for *T. gondii* while pregnant. Those mothers who were infected with *T. gondii* were more likely to show self-directed violence during the follow-up. The relative risk for death by suicide was 2.03, for violent suicide attempts 1.81, and for less violent suicide attempts 1.41, and a similar association was found for repetition of suicide attempts. The association was stronger in those mothers with no history of psychiatric disorder, and the risk of suicidal behavior increased with the level of the antibodies.

Zhang, et al. (2012) compared 54 adults who had attempted suicide with 30 normal controls and found that the attempted suicides were significantly more likely to be seropositive for *T. gondii*, even after controls for sex, age and body mass index, and the same association (although weaker) was found

[4] There were no sex differences, but non-white patients had higher levels of antibodies.
[5] The adjusted odds ratio was 1.57.

for *T. gondii* serointensity. No association was found between self-directed violence and other pathogens (cytomegalovirus and herpes simplex type 1).

One negative result has been published. Alvarado-Esquivel, et al. (2013) compared psychiatric outpatients in Mexico with a history of attempted suicide and those without such a history. There was no difference in the incidence of seropositivity for *T. gondii* (4.5% versus 7.9%, respectively). However, seropositively was more often higher than 150 IU/ml in the suicide attempters (100% of the seven attempters versus 50% of the ten non-suicidal outpatients). Those patients with current suicidal ideation also did not differ in the incidence of seropositivity from those without suicidal ideation.

Incidentally, Godwin (2012) suggested that high rate of suicide in veterinarians (Bartram and Baldwin, 2008) might be a result of their working with *T. gondii* infected animals (especially cats) in their practice, in addition to other factors such as stress, feelings of isolation, access to lethal drugs and desensitization to death through euthanizing animals.

Explanations for a Possible Association

Flegr (2013) noted that research indicates an association between *T. gondii* infections and a variety of problems, including traffic and workplace accidents and schizophrenia, as well as suicidal behavior. Research on the association of *T. gondii* with psychiatric disorders indicates that those seropositive for *T. gondii* are more likely to experience schizophrenia several years later, suggesting a cause-and-effect link for this association (Niebuhr, et al., 2007; Yolken and Torrey, 2008). Flegr noted that the brain morphology found to characterize schizophrenia as measured by MRIs is present only in schizophrenics who are *T. gondii* infected (Horacek, et al., 2012). Flegr also noted that, because *T. gondii* infections are present in about 30% of the worldwide population, the presence of a *T. gondii* infection is neither necessary nor sufficient to account for the appearance of schizophrenia or suicidal behavior.

Lafferty (2006) speculated that the mechanism for the association between national levels of neuroticism and the prevalence of *T. gondii* was that the parasite influenced the level of neurotransmitters such as dopamine, and Flegr (2013) concurred with this hypothesis.

Alternatively, research shows that men seropositive for *T. gondii* have higher levels of testosterone (Flegr, et al., 2008), and so testosterone may also mediate the link between *T. gondii* and suicidal behavior. Lester (1993, 2014) has suggested that testosterone may be responsible for the higher rate of violent suicidal behavior (defined by the method used for suicide – firearms and hanging versus an overdose of medication, for example) in men as compared to women. However, the link between *T. gondii* infections and increased levels of testosterone is found only in men and not in women (Flegr, et al., 2008).

Flegr (2013) noted that the mechanism linking *T. gondii* infection to suicidal behavior may also be mediated by the action of tryptophan which is an essential amino acid for many parasites, and Okusaga and Postolache (2012) noted that *T. gondii* infection may also affect kynurenine pathways in the brain[6] which are thought to mediate depression and, therefore, suicidal behavior.

Okusaga and Postolache noted that *T. gondii* infection is often localized in the amygdala which may reduce fear, and also in the prefrontal cortex which may reduce the ability to inhibit impulsive behavior. Both of these would increase the acquired capability to inflict self-harm, one of the three important variables resulting in suicidal behavior according to a new theory of suicide proposed by Joiner (2005).[7]

Flegr (2013) noted that *T. gondii* infection was associated with several other psychiatric disorders, including bipolar disorder, obsessive-compulsive disorder, and personality disorders, as well as medical disorders such as recurrent migraines and Parkinson disease, disorders that are risk factors for suicide. Furthermore, these associations may be even stronger in those born to mothers who already have a *T. gondii* infection. Webster, et al. (2006) hypothesized that the psychiatric medications for schizophrenia and mood disorders (such as bipolar affective disorder) may be effective because they inhibit the replication of *T. gondii* in the brain, and they found evidence to support this hypothesis using rats.

More generally, Thornhill and Fincher (2011), who found an association between national homicide rates and a general measure of the incidence of diseases caused by parasites, speculated that the stress from parasitic diseases leads to aggressive behaviors, increasing rates of homicide and child abuse.

---

[6] Kynurenine is a metabolite of the amino acid L-tryptophan.

[7] The other two variables are thwarted belongingness and perceived burdensomeness.

Comment

The association between *T. gondii* infection and suicidal behavior seems to be well-documented, and possible causal links for this association have been suggested and received some empirical support. It would be of great interest to explore whether *T. gondii* infection is associated also with other-directed violence (such as homicide) as well as self-directed violence. If an association between *T. gondii* infection and other–directed violence does exist, this would have an impact on our explanations for how *T. gondii* infection leads to self-directed violence. For example, it would suggest that *T. gondii* infection may impact impulsivity which in turn impacts both self-directed and other-directed violence.

The possible association between *T. gondii* infection and psychiatric disorders means that future research must control for the possible confounding variable of psychiatric disorder. It is important to ascertain whether the association between *T. gondii* infection and suicidal behavior is found in individuals who are free from psychiatric disorder as well as in those who have a psychiatric disorder. Future research on individuals should also examine the levels of the breakdown products of the major neurotransmitters in the cerebrospinal fluid at the same time as measuring the seropositivity and serointensity of *T. gondii.* Studies such as these would enable us to clarify the causal mechanism(s) at work in the link between suicidal behavior and *T. gondii* infection.

References

Alvarado-Esquivel, C., Sanchez-Anguiano, L. F., Arnaud-Gil, C. A., Lopez-Longoria, J. C., Molina-Espinoza, L. F., Estrada-Martinez, S., Liesenfeld, O., Hernandez-Tinoco, J., Sifuentes-Alvarez, A., and Salas-Martinez, C. (2013). *Toxoplasma gondii* infection and suicide attempts. *Journal of Nervous and Mental Disease,* 201, 948-952.

Arling, T. A., Yolken, R. H., Lapidus, M., Langenberg, P., Dickerson, F. B., Zimmerman, S. A., Balis, T., Cabassa, J. A., Scrandis, D. A., Tonelli, L. H., and Postolache, T. T. (2009). *Toxoplasma gondii* antibody titers and history of suicide attempts in patients with recurrent mood disorders. *Journal of Nervous and Mental Disease,* 197, 905-908.

Bartram, D. J. and Baldwin, D. S. (2008). Veterinary surgeons and suicide. *Veterinary Record,* 162(2), 36-40.

Flegr, J. (2013). How and why *Toxoplasma* makes us crazy. *Trends in Parasitology,* 29, 156-163.

Flegr, J., Lindová, J. and Kodym, P. (2008). Sex-dependent toxoplasmosis-associated differences in testosterone concentration in humans. *Parasitology,* 135, 427-431.

Godwin, R. (2012). *Toxoplasma gondii* and elevated suicide risk. *Veterinary Record,* 171(9), 225.

Horacek, J., Flegr, J., Tintera, J., Verebova, K., Spaniel, F., Novak, T., Brunovsky, M., Bubenikova-Valesova, V., Holub, D., Palenicek, T., and Höschl, C. (2012). Latent toxoplasmosis reduces gray matter density in schizophrenia bot not in controls. *World Journal of Biological Psychiatry,* 13, 501-509.

Joiner, T. E. (2005). *Why people die by suicide.* Cambridge, MA: Harvard University Press.

Kondrichin, S. and Lester, D. (1997). Finno-Ugrians and suicide. *Perceptual and Motor Skills,* 85, 514.

Lafferty, K. D. (2006). Can the common brain parasite, *Toxoplasma gondii,* influence human culture? *Proceedings of the Royal Society B, Biological Sciences,* 273, 2749-2755.

Lester, D. (1987). National distribution of blood groups, personal violence (suicide and homicide), and national character. *Personality and Individual Differences,* 8, 575-576.

Lester, D. (1993). Testosterone and suicide. *Personality and Individual Differences,* 15, 347-348.

Lester, D. (2010a). Brain parasites and suicide. *Psychological Reports,* 107, 424.

Lester, D. (2010b). Predicting European suicide rates with physiological indices. *Psychological Reports,* 107, 713-714.

Lester, D. (2012). *Toxoplasma gondii* and homicide. *Psychological Reports,* 111, 196-197.

Lester, D. (2014). The role of testosterone. In: D. Letser, J. F. Gunn and P. Quinnette (Eds.), *Suicide in men,* pp. 61-70. Springfield, IL: Charles C. Thomas.

Ling, V. J., Lester, D., Mortensen, P. M., Langenberg, P. W., and Postolache, T. T. (2011). *Toxoplasma gondii* seropositivity and suicide rates in women. *Journal of Nervous and Mental Disease,* 199, 440-444.

Niebuhr, D. W., Cowan, D. N., Millikan, A. M., Yolken, R., Li, Y., and Weber, N. (2007). Risk of schizophrenia and antibodies to *Toxoplasma gondii* among US military personnel. *Schizophrenia Bulletin,* 33, 243-244.

Okusaga, O., Langenberg, P., Sleemi, A., Vaswani, D., Giegling, I., Hartmann, A. M., Konte, B., Friedle, M., Groer, M. W., Yolken, R. H., Rujescu, D., and Postolache, T. T. (2011). *Toxoplasma gondii* antibody titers and history of suicide attempts in patients with schizophrenia. *Schizophrenia Research,* 133, 150-155.

Okusaga, O. and Postolache, T. T. (2012). *Toxoplasma gondii,* the immune system, and suicidal behavior. In: Y. Dwivedi (Ed.), *The neurological basis of suicide*, pp. 381-405. Boca Raton, FL: CRC Press.

Pedersen, M. G., Mortensen, P. B., Norgaard-Pedersen, B., and Postolache, T. T. (2012). *Toxoplasma gondii* infection and self-directed violence in mothers. *Archives of General Psychiatry,* 69, 1123-1130.

Thornhill, R. and Fincher, C. L. (2011). Parasite stress promotes homicide and child maltreatment. *Philosophical Transactions of the Royal Society B,* 366, 3466-3477.

Voracek, M. (2006). Suicide rate and national scores on the Big Five personality factors. *Perceptual and Motor Skills,* 102, 609-610.

Voracek, M. (2009). Big five personality factors and suicide rates in the United States. *Perceptual and Motor Skills,* 109, 208-212.

Webster, J. P., Lamberton, P. H. L., Donnelly, C. a., and Torrey, E. F. (2006). Parasites as causative agents of human affective disorders? *Proceedings of the Royal Society, B,* 273, 1023-1030.

Yagmur, F., Yazar, S., Temel, H. O., and Cavusoglu, M. (2010). May *Toxoplasma gondii* increase suicide attempt? *Forensic Science International,* 199, 15-17.

Yolken, R. H. and Torrey, E. F. (2008). Are some cases of psychosis caused by microbial agents? *Molecular Psychiatry,* 13, 470-479.

Zhang, Y., Träskman-Bendz, L., Janelidze, S., Langenberg, P., Saleh, A., Constantine, N., Okusaga, O., Bay-Richter, C., Brundin, L., and Postolache, T. T. (2012). *Toxoplasma gondii* immunoglobulin G antibodies and nonfatal suicidal self-directed violence. *Journal of Clinical Psychiatry,* 73, 1069-1076.

In: Recent Advances in Toxoplasmosis Research
Editor: Connor M. Lee
ISBN: 978-1-63117-914-3

Chapter 3

TOXOPLASMOSIS IN CATTLE

***Dulce Helena Camila dos Reis*[1], *Maerle Oliveira Maia*[1], *Juliana Ribeiro Sena Kefler*[1], *Alvimar José da Costa*[3], *Katia Denise Saraiva Bresciani*[2,3], *Klaus Casaro Saturnino*[1] and *Thaís Rabelo dos Santos*[1*]**

[1]Fundação Universidade Federal de Rondônia – UNIR, Departamento de Medicina Veterinária, Campus de Rolim de Moura, Rolim de Moura, Rondônia.
[2]UNESP, Universidade Estadual Paulista Júlio de Mesquita Filho, Faculdade de Medicina Veterinária de Araçatuba, Araçatuba, São Paulo.
[3]UNESP, Universidade Estadual Paulista Júlio de Mesquita Filho, Faculdade de Ciências Agrárias e Veterinárias, UNESP, Jaboticabal, São Paulo.

ABSTRACT

Bovines acquire Toxoplasma gondii mainly by congenital route and by ingestion of food or water containing oocysts, and soil contaminated with cat manure. These animals may be relatively resistant to infection, since the detection of cysts in their musculature is less frequent than in other species, despite being evidenced high occurrence of the parasite in serological surveys. In bovine the main means of prevention is the correct

---

* Corresponding author: rabelo.vet@hotmail.com.

storage of food and water without contact with the feces of cats. Humans are infected mainly by eating raw or undercooked bovine meat as well by ingestion of not pasteurized or boiled milk. Prophylaxis for a human being is to avoid the consumption of raw animal foods must be processed by baking, boiling or freezing, and the parasite is responsive to three if performed appropriately. In this context, new worldwide perspectives referring to means of transmission, clinical signs, diagnosis and treatments in cattle will be discussed.

INTRODUCTION

Toxoplasmosis is caused by the protozoan *Toxoplasma gondii* (Nicolle and Manceaux 1908; Splendore, 1908), which belongs to the phylum Apicomplexa, order Eucoccidiorida and family Sarcocystidae. First found in two countries in 1908. In Brazil by Splendore in July, from laboratory rabbits, and Nicolle and Manceaux, Tunisia - France, isolated forms derived from the rodent *Ctenodatylus gondii* (Frazao-Teixeira, 2006; Dubey, 2007). The name Toxon comes of the arc and plasma of the format, thus arc format was the first format of the morphological appearance of the parasite (Hill et al., 2006; Dubey, 2007). Gondii was the name given to the species of protozoan in 1909 by French researchers (Manceaux and Nicolle, 1908).

This parasite gets the attention for diversity and complexity of their life cycle (Dubey, 1994). It has three stages, or infective forms:

The oocyst: may differ in form and size according their development (Dubey et al., 1970). Of all stages of the the parasite life cycle is more resistant to the environment (Hill et al., 2006). Before sporulation, the oocysts are spherical and measure 10-12 mm in diameter, after sporulation, the oocyst becomes a sporocyst - infective form of the oocyst, this contains two sporozoites – infective form from the oocyst, this contains two sporozoites with size: 2 μm-6 μm until 2 μm-8 μm.

The tachyzoite: It has the form of a half moon, with this stage found by Nicolle and Manceaux in 1908 (Dubey, 1977, and 2007). Tachyzoites are responsible for the acute phase of the disease (da Silva, 2006), and this stage, the parasite also receives the name of trophozoite, agent capable of penetrating almost all cell in the body of the animal (Dubey, 2007).

The bradyzoites: is characteristic of slow multiplication. It was discovered in 1973 by Frenkel encysted in tissues so became known as cistozoíta. Nucleus present in the posterior region of the parasitic cell, which differs from other forms of development of the parasite - tachyzoites (Dubey, 1998; 2007).

The cats or other animals of the Felidae family eliminate *T. gondii* oocysts after ingesting infective any of the three forms (oocyte, tachyzoite and bradyzoites), Elmore, 2010.

The pre-patent period for the elimination of oocysts and the rate of elimination will depend on the infective form ingested by the definitive host. Thus, the prepatent to oocysts shedding period is 3-10 days, when the intake tissue cysts (bradyzoites), and 19 days or more occurs when there is ingestion of oocysts or tachyzoite (Dubey, 2007).

The rate of elimination of oocysts reduces almost by half when the cat, or other definitive host ingests tachyzoites, the elimination rate compared with ingestion of tissue cysts (Dubey, 2007). What should be related to the fact that the encysted forms are resistant to digestion by gastric juice, and the tachyzoites are destroyed so in touch with the same (Jacobs et al., 1960a), because the bradyzoites are coated by a double membrane - parasitophorous vacuole and cell membrane of the parasite - and thus resist the local pH.

The cycle then begins with the release of oocysts in the feces of cats, especially in the feces of the domestic cat. But contrary to what many think, this process occurs only once, usually after weaning, may occasionally be repeated (Dubey, 1986).

In the environment, this oocyst undergoes a change in its structure to become potentially infectious, and time this process influenced by temperature, humidity and concentration of environmental oxygen (Dubey, 1994; Hill et al. 2006.). The stage at which the oocysts eliminated in the feces infective stage spend - containing sporozoites - is called sporulation, and takes 1-5 days, depending on environmental conditions (Dubey & Beattie, 2000; Bowman, 2010). The oocysts are important tools for the dissemination of the parasite in the environment (SILVA et al., 2003), from where you can reach a large number and variety of intermediate hosts, and continue its life cycle.

When a warm blooded animals (mammal and bird) ingests sporulated oocyst through water, contaminated food, or through hand contact with the mouth, sporocyst ruptures in the intestine and releases the sporozoites in the epithelium. These fall in intestinal cells and lymph nodes yielding tachyzoites (Dubey. 1986; 1994; 2007). Tachyzoites travel through the blood and lymph, and can affect the cardiac muscles and skeletal muscles, in addition to the brain, liver, lymph nodes and other organs and tissues (Dubey, 1986). In the intermediate host perform asexual reproduction, where a tachyzoite divides and produces two with the same capacity, this process is specialized, and gets its name from binary fission (Smith, 2009; Dubey, 2007).

These forms suffer a reduction in their rate of multiplication, giving rise to colonies that later give rise to tissue cysts (Dubey, 1994; Smith, 2009). A single cyst can house up to hundreds of bradyzoites, characterizing the chronic or latent phase of toxoplasmosis (Dubey, 1994; Silva, 2006). The intermediate hosts carnivores become infected mainly through this stage of the parasite (Jacobs et al., 1960b). When they ingest containing tissue cysts, they undergo proteolytic enzymes of the stomach and intestine, which digest the wall of the cyst allowing the release of up to hundreds of bradyzoites in the intestinal lumen, which invade the enterocytes of the new host. In these cells, bradyzoites becomes again tachyzoites, which undergo rapid multiplication before another new tissue encystment (Dubey, 1986; 1994).

The conclusion and restart the cycle occurs when the cat ingests the three infectious forms. The ingestion of bradyzoites within tissue cysts also seems to be the most common source of infection in cats, making carnivorism primarily responsible for the continuity of the life cycle from intermediate hosts (Dubey, 2009). Occurs the action of gastric enzymes, as in other carnivores, resulting in the release of bradyzoites, which penetrate the intestinal cells, and lamina propria of the intestine of felines and multiply, forming tachyzoites (Hill et al., 2006), that pass through the phase of rapid multiplication.

In the cat the parasite performs both asexual reproduction (one tachyzoite that originates other two), as sexual, where male and female gametes unite to form the oocyst - gametogony (Hill et al., 2006; Dubey, 2007; Smith, 2009.). All this results in the release of millions of oocysts which are released into the intestinal lumen and excreted with the faeces of the felidae not form spores, or non-infectious (Dubey, 1986; 1994). In severe infection in felids, after ingestion of tissue cysts in the extra intestinal phase, or phase in which there is the formation of cysts in tissue can also occur (Dubey, 2007).

Sources of Infection

Faeces of cats infected with *T. gondii* oocysts contaminate food, water and environment, leading to contamination of other animals through the ingestion of these sites present (Dubey & Beattie, 2000) oocysts. In animals with primary care is the contamination of feed, hay and silage by feces of infected with oocyst cat, but the contamination of pastures may also occur in animals Extensive creations (Albuquerque et al., 2011). Or transmission occur mechanically by invertebrates: flies, cockroaches, beetles, and worms that can spread oocysts in food for humans and animals (Hill et al., 2006.).

In other animals toxoplasmosis is almost an asymptomatic, manifestations and clinical signs depend on the nutritional and physiological state of the animal; infecting strain and place of formation of cysts. The signs are not specific toxoplasmosis besides insufficient for definitive diagnosis, because it resembles several other diseases (Costa et al., 1977; Hill et al., 2006).

For humans the most common ways of infection is by the oral route, occurring with eating raw or undercooked meat containing cysts of Toxoplasma, ingestion of oocysts present in sandboxes, unwashed vegetables and contaminated water, and less common contamination by ingestion of tachyzoites present in raw milk (goat or cow), breast milk, saliva of animals by licking, sperm or through laboratory accidents (Dubey & Beattie, 2000; Dubey & Jones, 2008). Another means of transmission of *T. gondii* is via the placenta, which happens when non-immune hosts are infected during pregnancy. The parasite proliferates in the placenta and reaches the fetus, leading to irreversible miscarriages or congenital lesions. Infection can also occur by blood transfusion and organ transplantation, but contains the same meaning as the ingestion of infected tissues (Dubey, 1994; Lindsay, 2007).

TOXOPLASMOSIS

It is a disease caused by *Toxoplasma gondii*, which refers to an enteric coccidia in domestic cat, or other members of the family Filidae (Bowman, 2010). It is a disease of great worldwide distribution, with rates that can vary from 0 to 99% in humans, domestic and wild animals. Being found in many different species of domestic and wild animals in all regions of the world, in various climates, topography and socioeconomic conditions (Dubey & Beattie, 2000; Ministry of Health, 2004; Dubey, Lindsay, 2007).

Like other mammals, the human being is also an intermediate host for *T. gondii*, toxoplasmosis classified as a zoonosis. In humans the pathogenesis of the disease is highly variable, as are many factors that define the appearance of the disease and its clinical manifestations, such as strain, route of infection; volume of infective forms and finally the immune status the host (Dubey & Beattie, 2000; Meneo & Kawazoe, 2011). Thus toxoplasmosis can manifest from a fever with lymph node infarction, will seriously injure the central nervous system, retina and myocardium (Dubey and Jones, 2008; Ministry of Health, 2004).

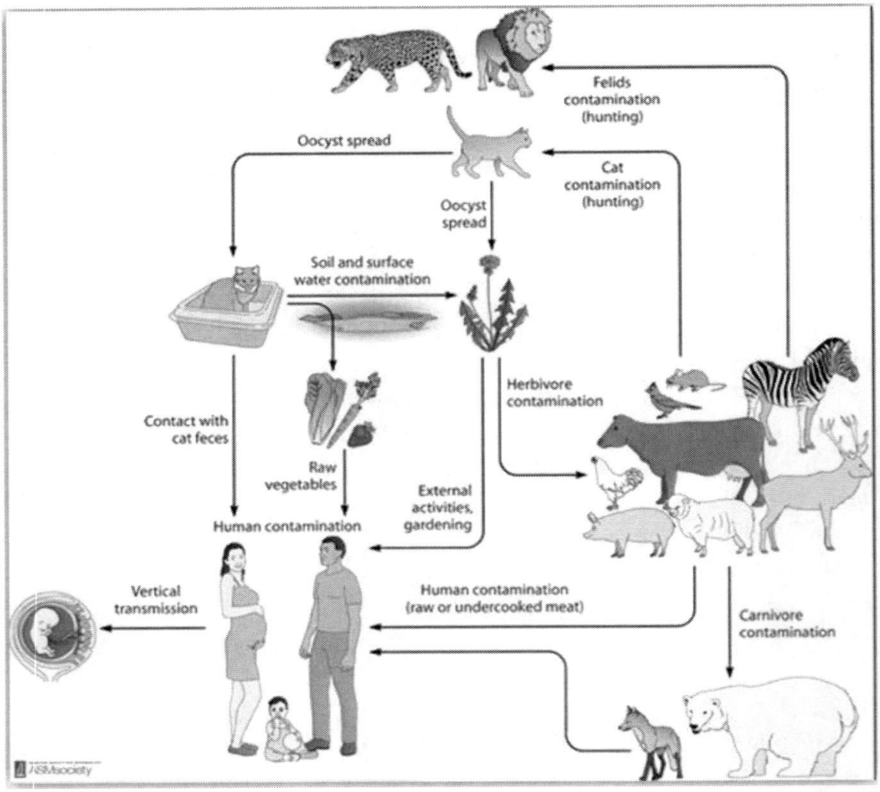

Figure 1. Cycle of *Toxoplasma gondii*, with its various forms of infection for humans (ASM).

The lesions of congenital transmission showed greater severity in the fetus and newborn, and are characterized by encephalitis, jaundice, rash and hepatomegaly, which may or may not be associated with chorioretinitis, hydrocephalus, and microcephaly, with high rates of morbidity and mortality (Dubey, 1986; Dubey & Beattie, 2000; Meneo & Kawazoe, 2011). Besides these known symptoms in humans caused by the parasite, studies seek clarification of a possible change in behavior that causes toxoplasmosis in humans and in animals (Bech-Nielsen, 2011).

TOXOPLASMOSIS IN CATTLE

In 2011, the cattle according to the Department of Agriculture of the United States - USDA, is around 1.01 billion animals, Excelling in countries with larger herd India, Brazil, United States and China. Beef is the third most consumed worldwide, being the main source of animal protein in Africa and Oceania (ROPPA, 2009; OECD and FAO, 2013). The most prominent consumer the United States, Australia and Brazil (ANALPEC, 2006).

As with other domestic animals, cattle can also be infected with *T. gondii*, usually related to the presence of cat feces and water or food (Albuquerque et al., 2011), also making them one of the intermediate hosts of the parasite . The natural disease in cattle was first diagnosed in Germany in 1952 by Houesdorf & Holtz (Mayer, 1965; Costa et al., 1977; Oliveira, 1997), and Ohio in the United States (Dubey & Beattie, 2000). And the first experimental oral inoculation of oocysts in cattle was carried out by Costa et al., 1977, in São Paulo - Brazil.

Since then it has become common in experiments which use the oral form of infection, to evaluate symptoms and isolation of cysts as well as regarding the transmission of the parasite through this domestic species (Dubey, 1983; Esteban-Redondo & Innes, 1997; Esteban Redondo et al., 1999). Works with prevalence of anti-Toxoplasma antibodies in cattle, as in other domestic species are increasingly common around the world, where rates ranging from 0 to 76% prevalence, illustrated in Table 1 are found.

The frequency of *T. gondii* infection in cattle is significant, which suggests that these animals represent an important source of contamination for humans (Costa et al., 1977; Santos et al., 2009), is of great importance in Public Health (Silveira, 2002). According to Dubey (1983; 2000), the *T. gondii* cysts can remain viable in bovine tissues for several days after infection, reaching the age of slaughter of these animals. However, although they may be contaminated with success, cattle are considered "bad" host for *T. gondii*, it seem to have a natural resistance to the parasite, where it is eliminated or reduced to undetectable levels within a few weeks after infection (Dubey, 1983, 1986; Dubey & Jones, 2008; Hill & Dubey, 2013) and had a lower number of cysts in the muscle compared to other species (Dubey, 1994)

Table 1. Occurrence (%) of antibodies against *Toxoplasma gondii* in cattle from different countries, their respective outores, number of animals and techniques

Country	State/ Region	Author	Number of examined animals	Techniques	Occurrence (%)
Brazil	Paraná	Marana et al., 1994	334	RIFI	32, 3%
		Marana et al., 1995	503	RIFI	48,5%
		Garcia et al., 1999	400	RIFI	25, 8%
		Daguer et al., 2004	348	RIFI	41, 4%
		Ogawa et al., 2005	385	RIFI	26,0%
	Rio de Janeiro	Albuquerque et al., 2005	589	RIFI	14,8%
		Frazão-Teixeira, 2006	77	ELISA	49,5%
		Luciano et al., 2011	459	RIFI	2,0%
	São Paulo	Costa et al., 2001	506	RIFI	55,3%
		Silveira, 2002	638	RIFI	34,8%-
		Meireles, 2003	200	ELISA	11,0%
	Minas Gerais	Costa and Costa, 1978		RIFI	12,0%
		Passos et al., 1984		RIFI	9,0%
		Costa et al., 2001	94	RIFI	16,0%
	Pará	Carmo et al., 2010	500	RIFI	40,6%
	Mato Grosso	Santos et al., 2009	2000	RIFI	71,0%
	Mato Grosso do Sul	Araújo et al., 1998		-	4,3%
	Amazônia	Ferraroni e Marzochi, 1980	25	RHAI	60,0%
	Bahia	Oliveira et al., 2001		RIFI	9,8%
		Godin et al., 1999		LAT	1,0%
Portugal	North	Lopes et al., 2013	161	MAT	7,5%
Malaysia	Selagor	Normaznah et al.	73	IFAT	3,8%
Iran	-	Hashemi-Fesharki, 1995	2000	LAT	0,0%
	Tabri	Nematollahi and Moghddam, 2008	490	IFAT	15,9%
	Kerman	Sanati et al., 2012	300	MAT	71,3%
Serbia	-	Klun et al., 2006	611	MAT	76,3%
Sudan	-	Elfahal et al., 2013	181	ELISA	13,3%

Clinical toxoplasmosis in cattle is rare, and abortions are uncommon, however the physiological disorders are more evident in taurine compared to zebu cattle and buffalo, as well as the title of highest anti-Toxoplasma antibodies (Olivera, 1997). Not to mention that attempts to isolate *T. gondii* tissue in cattle are often unsuccessful, indicating the meat of these animals as a means of transmission unimportant, relative to other domestic animals (Jacobs & Cols, 1960b; Zardi & Cols, 1964; Mayer, 1967, Work 1967, Qatar & Cols, 1969; Jamra & Cols, 1969; Oliveira, 1997; Dubey, 2007; Lindsay, 2007; Dubey & Jones, 2008)

The congenital transmission resulting in abortions, and vertical transmission can occur, similar to neosporosis form but is rare (Moore et al., 2008; Wiengcharoen et al., 2011), thus characterizing the neosporosis for causing abortions in cattle by protozoáriao. In an experiment with 50 cows, of these , 18 % (9) were positive for toxoplasmosis , but the calves born only 3 of them also have positive titers (Costa et al., 2011) . In the study by Santos et al., 2009, there was some association with abortion of cows in the last 12 months, with the high rate of seroprevalence for toxoplasmosis. Compared to cow's milk when compared to goat milk is an important source of infection of toxoplasmosis in humans (Jones et al. , 2009) , it is believed that there is little or no risk of infection by *T. gondii* cow's milk drink , which is normally pasteurized or cooked (Hill et al., 2006; Costa et al., 2011) , however , the risk of toxoplasmosis infection is real when it is fresh milk or food in which milk is not processed (Hiramoto et al., 2001).

In cattle the most widely used diagnostic methods are ELISA - Enzyme immunoassay and IFA - Reaction indirect immunofluorescence, but the modified agglutination test (MAT) also seems to be indicative of *T. gondii* infection in cattle (Dubey et al., 1985; Dubey & Jones, 2008). The latter was developed in 1965 by Fulton, improved in 1980 by Desmonts and Remington and Dubey and Desmonts in 1987, used as diagnostics in animals (Dubey, 2007). One of methods of molecular diagnostics, PCR can also be used as a diagnostic method in animals (Bastien, 2002). This diagnostic consists of a chain reaction of polymerase enzyme, using the DNA of the agent (Dubey, 2007).

It is widely used in surveys which seeks cysts in tissues of slaughtered animals, and retail meats available (Hill et al., 2006;. Dubey, 2007; Opsteegh et al., 2010; Santos et al., 2010). Since the identification of the parasite in tissue is limited in other tests due to sample size (Costa et al., 2011). Other methods are also known latex agglutination (LAT) and Immunosorbent Assay (IAAT) Hill et al. 2006. Some commonly used for other species, methods may exhibit erratic results with sera from cattle (Dubey et al., 1985), especially in naturally infected animals. An example is the test Sabeim Feldaman-1948, or dye testing, using highly sensitive and specific dye for toxoplasmosis. To detect very low titers of toxoplasmosis in humans (Dubey, 2007).

Treatment, Control and Prevention

In humans, treatment consists in the use of sulfonamide associated with pyrimethamine. The esperimetamina is also used in particular as a prophylactic means in pregnant women because they are not toxic and will not cross the placenta. Serological screening during pregnancy is very important Paw reducing congenital toxoplasmosis, characterized in France in 1960 (Dubey, 2007).

Should avoid the exchange of shares of Sand by pregnant women (Hill et al., 2006), cash and have them deleted in safe waste. Avoid the use of products of animal origin raw or undercooked (Hiramoto et al., 2001), *T. gondii* is killed in exposed to extreme heat or cold tissue in prolonged heat, so one should not taste the food during cooking and wash hands after handling raw meat or contaminated land (Tenter et al., 2000; Ministry of Health, 2004). And there is no human vaccine for Toxoplasma (Dubey, 2007).

In animals, especially cattle, prevention is for the care and storage of the grain silo, without contact with these foods faeces of domestic cats (Santos et al., 2009). An oral vaccine comprising live bradyzoites, has been effective to prevent release of oocysts in cats, however the duration of protective immunity is not yet well established, and is not yet available on the market (Kijlstra & Jongert, 2008).

Conclusion

Toxoplasmosis is an enteric Coccidial domestic cat, caused by the protozoan *Toxoplasma gondii*, the phylum Apicomplexa, which has three infective forms (oocysts, tachyzoites and bradizoíto). Can infect human and animals by the ingestion of one infectious form, in particular oocysts present in food and water in the case of herbivorous animals and humans. Or infection may occur via the placenta, which acquire more severe in fetuses and newborns. The cattle are one of the most used protein sources in the world, and is also an intermediate host for toxoplasmosis. However, it is a smaller transmitter, because these animals have a natural resistance, or reduce the parasite indetáveis levels, transmission by milk is insignificant when compared to other species such as goats, the occurrence of abortions are rare It is more common abortion caused by protozoan Neospora caninum. Even when dealing with a smaller transmitter, cattle can remain long with the cysts of the parasite in their tissues, and the high seroprevalence in cattle worldwide is a concern for public health. The farm animals are not treated against zoonosis, getting treatment based on the use of sulfa drugs and other chemotherapeutic agents for use in humans and companion animals. In these animals the main means of prevention is the correct storage of food and water without contact with the feces of cats. Prophylaxis for a human being is to avoid the consumption of raw animal foods must be processed by baking, boiling or freezing, and the parasite is responsive to three if performed appropriately.

References

Albuquerque, GR; Munhoz, AD; Flausino, W; Silva, RT; Almeida, CRR; Medeiros, SM; Lopes, CWG. Prevalência de anticorpos anti-*Toxoplasma gondii* em bovinos leiteiros do vale do paraíba sul fluminense, estado do Rio de Janeiro. *Rev. Bras. Parasitol. Vet.*, v.14, n.3, 25-128, 2005.

Albuquerque, GR; Munhoz, AD; Teixeira, M; Flausino, W; Medeiros, SM; Lopes, CW. Risk factors associated with *Toxoplasma gondii* infection in dairy cattle, State of Rio de Janeiro. *Pesq. Vet. Bras*, v. 31, 287-290, Rio de Janeiro, 2011.

Araújo, FR; Carvalho, CME; Balbuena, CB. levantamento sorológico para *Toxoplasma gondii*em bovinos de corte do Estado de Mato Grosso do Sul, Brasil. *Revista Brasileira de Medicina Veterinária*, v. 20, n. 5, 201-203, 1998.

ASM, 2013. Disponível em: http://cmr.asm.org/content/25/2/264.figures-only ology.html Acesso em 14 de dezembro de 2011. 12 de Fevereiro de 2014.

Bastien, P. Diagnosis: Molecular diagnosis of toxoplasmosis. *Transations of the royal society of tropical medicina and hygiene*, v. 96, 2002.

Bech-Nielsen, S. *Toxoplasma gondii* associated behavioural changes in mice, rats and humans: Evidence from current research. *Preventive Veterinary Medicine*, 103, 78–79, 2012.

Bowman, DD. Gorgis: Parasitologia Veterinária. Publishing house: Elsevier, Rio de Janeiro, 2010.

Brazil. Ministério da Saúde. Fundação Nacional de Saúde. Doenças Infecciosas e Parasitárias. 4ª Edição, Brasília, 2004.

Carmo, EL; Neves, CS; Marinho, RR; Silva, AV; Lima, MS; Moraes, CCG; Póvoa, MM. Inquérito sorológico para *Toxoplasma gondii* em bovinos abatidos na região metropolitana de Belém, PA. 2010.

Costa, AJ; Araujo, FG; Costa, JO; Lima, JD; Nascimento, E. Experimental infection of bovines with oocysts of *Toxoplasma gondii. J. Parasitol.*, v.63, n.2, 212-214, 1977.

Costa, AJ; Costa, EP. frequência de bovinos reagentes à reação de Imunoflourescencia Indireta para *Toxoplasma gondii* em Poços de Caldas, MG, Brasil. *Arquivos da Escola de Veterinária da UFMG*, Belo Horizonte, v. 30, n. 1, 47-51, 1978.

Costa, GHN; Costa, AJ da; Lopes, WDZ; Bresciani, KDS; Santos, TR dos; Esper, CR, Santana, ÁE. *Toxoplasma gondii*: Infection natural congenital in cattle and an experimental inoculation of gestating cows with oocysts. *Experimental Parasitology*, v.127, 277–281, 2011.

Daguer, H; Vicente, RT; Costa, T; Virmond, MP; Hamann, W; Amendoeira, MR. Soroprevalência de anticorpos anti-*Toxoplasma gondii* em bovinos e funcionários de matadouros da microrregião de Pato Branco, Paraná, Brasil. *Ciência Rural*, v.34, n.4, 1133-1137, 2004.

Dubey, JP; Beattie, CP. Toxoplasmosis of Animals and Man. Publishing house: *Boca Raton*, Flórida, 2000.

Dubey, JP. Advances in the life cycle of *Toxoplasma gondii. International Journal for Parasitology*, 28: 1019-24, 1998.

Dubey, JP. Distribution of cysts and tachyzoites in calves and pregnant cows inoculated with *Toxoplasma gondii* oocysts. *Veterinary Parasitology*, 13, 199-211. 1983.

Dubey, JP. History of the discovery of the life cycle of *Toxoplasma gondii. International Journal for Parasitology*, v.39, 877-882, 2009.

Dubey, JP. The History and Life Cycle of *Toxoplasma gondii. Toxoplasma gondii.* The Model Apicomplexan – Perspectives and Methods. Publishing house: Elsevier, 2007a.

Dubey, JP. Toxoplasma, Hammondia, Besnoitia, Sarcocystis and other tissue cyst-forming coccidian of man and animals. In: KREIER, *J. P. Parasitic Protozoa.* Gregarines, Haemogregarines, Coccidia, Plasmodia and Haemoproteids, v. 3, Nova Iorque: Academic Press, 563 p, 1977.

Dubey, JP. Toxoplasmosis. *Journal of the American Veterinary Medical Association*, 205, 1593-8. 1994

Dubey, JP. Serologic prevalence of toxoplasmosis in cattle, sheep, goats, pigs, bison, and elk in Montana. *J. Am. Vet. Med. Assoc.*, 186, 969–970, 1985.

Dubey, JP. Toxoplasmosis. *J. Am. Vet. Med. Assoc.*, 189, 166-170, 1986.

Dubey, JP; Jones, JL. *Toxoplasma gondii* infection in humans and animals in the United States. *International Journal for Parasitology*, v. 38, 1257–1278, 2008.

Dubey, JP; Miller, NL; Frenkel, JK. Characterization of the new fecal form of *Toxoplasma gondii*. *J. Parasitol.*, 56, 447–456, 1970.

Elfahal, AM; Elhassan, AM; Hussien, MO; Enan, KA; Musa, AB; El Hussein, AM. Seroprevalence of *Toxoplasma gondii* in Dairy Cattle with Reproductive Problems in Sudan. *ISRN Veterinary Science*, 4p, 2013.

Elmore, SA; Jones, JL; Conrad, PA; Patton, S; Lindsay, DS; Dubey, JP. *Toxoplasma gondii*: epidemiology, feline clinical aspects, and prevention. *Trends in Parasitology*, v.26, n. 4, 191-196, 2010.

Estaban-Redondo, I; Innes, EA. *Toxoplasma gondii* infection in sheep and cattle. *Comp. Immun. Microbiol.*, v. 20, n.2, 191-196, Elsevier Science, 1997.

Esteban-Redondo, I; Maley, SW; Thomson, K; Nicoll, S; Wright, S; Buxton, D; Innes, EA. Detection of *T. gondii* in tissues of sheep and cattle following oral infection. *Veterinary Parasitology*, v.86, 155–171, 1999.

Ferraroni, JJE; Marzochi, MC. Prevalence of *Toxoplasma gondii* infection in domestic and wild animals, and human groups of the Amazonas region. *Memórias do Instituto Oswaldo Cruz.*, v.75, n.1-2, 99-109, 1980.

Frazão-Teixeira, E. Toxoplasmose em bovinos e suínos, e a viabilidade de cistos de *Toxoplasma gondii* em encéfalos suínos no município de Campos dos Goytacazes/ RJ. 2006. 97f. Dissertação (Mestrado em Medicina Veterinária – área de concentração: Produção Animal) – Centro de Ciências e Tecnologias Agropecuárias, UENF, Campos dos Goytacazes, RJ, 2006.

Garcia, JL; Navarro, IT; Ogawa, L; Oliveira, RC. Soroprevalência do *Toxoplasma gondii* em suínos, bovinos, ovinos e eqüinos, e sua correlação com humanos, felinos e caninos, oriundos de propriedades rurais do norte do Paraná, Brasil. *Ciência Rural*, v. 29, n. 01, 91-97, 1999.

Godim, LFP; Sartor, IF; Hasegawa, M; et al. Sororpevalencia of Neospora caninum in dairy cattle in Bahia, Brazil. *Veterinary Parasitology*, Amisterdan, v. 86, 71-75, 1999.

Hashemi-Fesharki, R. Seroprevalence of *Toxoplasma gondii* in cattle, sheep and goats in Iran. *Veterinary Parasitology*, v.61, n.1-2, 1-3, 1996.

Hill, DE; Chirukandoth, S; Dubey, JP. Biology and epidemiology of *Toxoplasma gondii* in man and animals. *Animal Health Research Reviews*, 6 (1), 41–61, 2005.

Hill, DE; Dubey, JP. *Toxoplasma gondii* prevalence in farm animals in the United States. *International Journal for Parasitology*, v.43, 107–113, 2013.

Hiramoto, RM; Mayrbaurl-Borges, M; Galisteo Júnior, AJ; Meireles, LR; Macre, MS; Andrade Junior, HF. Infectivity of cysts of the ME-49 *Toxoplasma gondii* strain in bovine milk and homemade cheese. *Rev Saúde Pública*, v.35, 113-118, 2001.

Jacobs, L; Remington, JS; Melton, ML. A survey of meat samples from swine, cattle, and sheep for the presence of encysted Toxoplasma. *J. Parasitol*, 46, 23–28, 1960b.

Jacobs, L; Remington, JS; Melton, ML. The resistance of the encysted form of *Toxoplasma gondii. J. Parasitol*, 46, 11–21, 1960a.

Kijlstra, A; Jongert, E. Control of the risk of human toxoplasmosis transmitted by meat. *International Journal for Parasitology*, 38, 1359–1370, 2008.

Klun, I; Djakovic, OD; Radivojevic, SK; Nikolic, A. Cross-sectional survey on *Toxoplasma gondii* infection in cattle, sheep and pigs in Serbia: Seroprevalence and risk factors. *Veterinary Parasitology*, v.135, 121–131, 2006.

Lindsay, DS; Dubey, JP. Toxoplasmosis in Wild and Domestic Animals. *Toxoplasma gondii. The Model Apicomplexan – Perspectives and Methods*. Publishing house: Elsevier, 2007.

Lopes, AP; Dubey, JP; Neto, F; Rodrigues, A; Martinsd, T; Rodrigues, M; Cardoso, L. Seroprevalence of Toxoplasma gondii infection in cattle, sheep, goats and pigs from the North of Portugal for human consumption. *Veterinary Parasitology*, 193, 266– 269, 2013.

Luciano, DM; Menezes, RC; Ferreira, LC; Nicolau, JL; Neves, LB das; Luciano, RM; Dahroug, MAA; Amendoeira, MRR. Occurrence of anti-*Toxoplasma* gondii antibodies in cattle and pigs slaughtered, State of Rio de Janeiro. *Rev. Bras. Parasitol. Vet.*, Jaboticabal, v. 20, n. 4, 351-353, 2011.

Marana, ERM; Navarro, IT; Vidotto, O; Freire, RL; Lott, R. Ocorrência de anticorpos anti-*Toxoplasma gondii* em bovinos de corte, abatidos em matadouros do norte do Paraná - Brasil. *Semina: Ciências Agrárias*, v.15, n.1, 38-40, 1994.

Marana, ERM; Venturini, ACH; Freire, RL. Ocorrência de anticorpos anti-*Toxoplasma gondii* em rebanhos de bovinos de leite do norte do Paraná - Brasil. *Semina: Ciências Agrárias*, v.16, n.1, 40-42, Mar. 1995.

Mayer, HF. Investigaciones sobre toxoplasmosis. *Bol. Of. Sant. Panam.*, v. 58, n.6, 485-497, 1965.

Meireles, LR; Galisteo Jr, AJ; Andrade Jr, HF. Serological survey of antibodies to *Toxoplasma gondii* in food animals from São Paulo state, Brazil. *Brazilian Journal of Veterinary Research and Animal Science*, v.40, 267-271, 2003.

Moore, DP; Regidor-Cerrillo, J; Morrell, E; Poso, MA; Cano, DB; Leunda, MR; Linschinky, L Odéon, AC; Odriozola, E; Ortega-Mora, LM; Campero, CM. The role of *Neospora caninum* and *Toxoplasma gondii* in spontaneous bovine abortion in Argentina. *Veterinary Parasitology*, v.156, 163–167, 2008.

Nematollahi, A; Moghddam, GH. Survey on Seroprevalence of Anti-*Toxoplasma Gondii* Antibodies in Cattle in Tabriz (Iran) by IFAT. *American Journal of Animal and Veterinary Sciences*, v. 3, 40-42, 2008.

Nicolle, C; Manceaux, L. (1909). Sur un protozoaire nouveau du gondi. *C. R. Seances Acad. Sci.*, 148, 369–372.

Normanznah, Y; Saniah, K; Fuzina, N; Naseem, M; Khatijah, M. Prevalence of antibodies to Toxoplasma gondii among farmers and cattle in Gombak District, Selangor, Malaysia. A Preliminary Report. *Tropical Biomedicine*, 2004. v.21, 157-159.

Ogawa, L; Freire, RL; Vidotto, O; Gondim, LFP; Navarro, IT. Occurrence of antibodies to Neospora caninum and *Toxoplasma gondii* in dairy cattle from the northern region of the Paraná State, Brazil *Arq. Bras. Med. Vet. Zootec.*, v.57, n.3, 2005.

Oliveira, LMGB; Oliveira, AMWA; Azevedo, SJ; Oréfice, F. Toxoplasmosis in southeastern Brazil: an alarming situation of highly endemic acquired and congenital infection. In: PETERSON E, POLLAK A, OWONA IR. Recent trends in research on congenital toxoplasmosis. *Intern. J. Parasitol.*, v.31, 115-44, 2001.

Oliveira, FCR. Infecção experimental de *Bos taurus*, *Bos indicus* e *Bubalus buvalis* com oocisto de *Toxoplasma gondii.* Estudo comparativo. 1997. 92f. Dissertação (Mestrado em Patologia Animal) – Faculdade de Ciências Agrárias e Veterinárias, Universidade Estadual Paulista, Jaboticabal, 1997.

Oliveira, LMGB; Oliveira, AMWA; Azevedo, SJ; Oréfice , F. Toxoplasmosis in southeasttern Brazil: na alarming situatoin of highly endemic acquired and congenital infection. In PETERSON E, POLLAK A, OWONA IR. Recent trends in rearch on congenital toxoplasmosis. *Internacional Journal of Parasitology*, v. 31, 15-44, 2001.

Onyiche, TE; Ademola, IO. (2013) Seroprevalence of anti-*Toxoplasma gondii* antibodies in cattle and pigs in Ibadan, Nigeria. *Journal of Parasitic Diseases.*

Passos, LMF; Lima, JD; Figueiredo, BL. Determinação da infecção por *Toxoplasma gondii* em bovinos abatidos em Belo Horizonte (MG) através da frequência de anticorpos e tentativa de isolamento a partir de musculatura diafragmática. *Arquivos Brasileiros de Medicina Veterinária e Zootecnia*, v. 36, n. 5, 581-589, 1984.

Sanati, H; Fard, SRN; Nahrevanian, H; Khalili, M; Safari, Z. Seroprevalence of Toxoplasma gondiiAntibodies in Dairy Cows in Kerman Province, South East Iran. *Current Research Journal of Biological Sciences*, 4, 417-421, 2012.

Santos, SL; Costa, KS; Gondim, LQ; Silva, MSA; Uzêda, RS; Abe-Sandes, K; Gondim, LFP. Investigation of *Neospora caninum*, *Hammondia* sp., and *Toxoplasma gondii* in tissues from slaughtered beef cattle in Bahia, Brazil. *Parasitol Res.*, 106, 457–461, 2010.

Santos, TR; Costa, AJ; Toniollo, GH; Luvizotto, MCR; Benetti, AH; Santos, RR; Matta, DH; Lopes, WDZ; Oliveira, JA; Oliveira, GP. Prevalence of anti-*Toxoplasma gondii* antibodies in dairy cattle, dogs, and humans from the Jauru micro-region, Mato Grosso state, Brazil. *Veterinary Parasitology*, 161, 324–326, 2009.

Silva, RC. da. Diferenciação entre os estágios agudo e crônico na infecção toxoplásmica pela técnica de aglutinação direta modificada. Dissertação (Mestrado em Medicina Veterinária) – Universidade Estadual Paulista, Faculdade de Medicina Veterinária e Zootecnia, Botucatu, 2006.

Silva, S; Bahia-Oliveira, LM; Shen, SK; Kwok, OC; Lehman, T; Dubey, JP. Prevalence of *Toxoplasma gondii* in chickens from an area in southern Brazil highly endemic to humans. *The Journal of Parasitology*, 89, 394-6, 2003.

Silveira, DM. *Pesquisa de anticorpo contra Neospora caninum e Toxoplasma gondii em bovinos leiteiros da região nordeste de São Paulo***.** 2002. 62f. Dissertaçã (Mestrado em Medicina Veterinária) – Faculdade de Ciências Agrárias e Veterinárias, Universidade Estadual Paulista, Jaboicabal, 2002.

Smith, JE. Tracking Transmission of the Zoonosis *Toxoplasma gondii*. *Advances in Parasitology*, v. 68, 139-159. Publishing house: Elsevier, 2009.

Splendore, A. Un nuovo protozoa parassita de'conigli. incontrato nelle lesioni anatomiche d'une malattia che ricorda in molti punti il Kala-azar dell'uomo. *C. R. Seances Acad. Sci.*, 147,763–766, 1908.

Tenter, AM; Heckeroth, AR; Weiss, LM. *Toxoplasma gondii*: from animals to humans. *International Journal for Parasitology*, 30, 1217-1258, 2000.

Wiengcharoen, J; Thompson, RCA; Nakthong, C; Rattanakorn, P; Sukthana, Y. Transplacental transmission in cattle: is *Toxoplasma gondii* less potent *than Neospora caninum*?. *Parasitol Res.*, V.108, 1235–1241, 2011.

In: Recent Advances in Toxoplasmosis Research ISBN: 978-1-63117-914-3
Editor: Connor M. Lee

Chapter 4

TOXOPLASMOSIS IN GOATS

Lucas Shigaki de Matos[1*], Julia Cestari Pierucci[1], Luiz da Silveira Neto[1], Lucilene Granuzzio Camossi[2], Daniel Fontana Ferreira Cardia[2], Alvimar José da Costa[1], Thais Rabelo dos Santos[4] and Katia Denise Saraiva Bresciani[1,3]

[1]UNESP, Universidade Estadual Paulista Julio de Mesquita Filho, Faculdade de Ciências Agrárias e Veterinárias, Jaboticabal, São Paulo.
[2]UNESP, Universidade Estadual Paulista Júlio de Mesquita Filho, Faculdade de Medicina Veterinária e Zootecnia de Botucatu, Botucatu, São Paulo.
[3]UNESP, Universidade Estadual Paulista Julio de Mesquita Filho, Faculdade de Medicina Veterinária de Araçatuba, Araçatuba, São Paulo.
[4]UNIR, Fundação Universidade Federal de Rondônia, Departamento de Medicina Veterinária, Campus de Rolim de Moura, Rolim de Moura, Rondônia

ABSTRACT

Toxoplasma gondii is the etiologic agent of a worldwide distribution zoonosis. Cats are denominated as definitive hosts, but the infection affects many species including goats. Ingestion of oocysts excreted in

[*] Email: lucasvsm@hotmail.com

definitive hosts feces, as well as water and soil, and via the transplacental represents the source of contamination. Goats infected with *T. gondii* will develop fever, anorexia, dyspnea, and pregnant females, in addition to those mentioned signs, will suffer miscarriage and stillbirth. Therefore this chapter will discuss relevant topics on the epidemiology, clinical signs, diagnosis, treatment and control of this disease so important and widespread in the world.

INTRODUCTION

Toxoplasmosis is an important cause of high morbidity and mortality in immunocompromised individuals and can also lead to serious health problems in healthy adults (Luft et al., 1993; Montoya and Liesenfeld, 2004), being considered the etiological agent of a cosmopolitan character zoonosis and with marked medical and veterinary importance (Tzanidakis et al., 2012).

The protozoan *Toxoplasma gondii* has a facultative heteroxenous life cycle and affects warm-blooded animals, including terrestrial and marine mammals, birds and humans (Dubey, 2009), causing abortion and congenital diseases in various species of intermediate hosts, in particular goats (Tenter et al., 2000; Dubey, 2010).

The world`s goat herd consists of 807.6 million heads and the meat production is estimated at 4.5 million tons (FAO, 2010). Of that total, Brazil has about 14 million animals (IBGE, 2013) being this activity economically important in the country. Such activity stands out due to the relevant animal derived products such as meat, milk, wool and fur. The dairy goat production is estimated at 21 million liters/year and involves, mostly, small companies (MAPA, 2014).

Toxoplasmosis has been incriminated as a major cause of reproductive problems in sheep and goats in United States (Dubey and Beattie, 1988), Norway (Skjerve et al., 1998), Uruguay (Freyre et al., 1999), Ghana (Van Der Puije et al., 2000), Tobago (Borde et al., 2006), China (Wang et al., 2011), Romania (Lovu et al., 2012), Portugal (Lopes et al., 2013), Iran (Bayat et al., 2013) and Ethiopia (Gebremedhin et al., 2013).

Investigations on animal toxoplasmosis are essential due to its transmission to humans and their pathogenicity in production animals (Hill and Dubey, 2013; Lopes et al., 2013; Anastasia et al., 2013; Esquivel et al., 2013; Juránková et al., 2014)

History of Toxoplasmosis in Goats

The first record of *T. gondii* was stablished in 1908 by Nicolle and Manceaux from a liver sample of a rodent denominated *Ctnodactylus gundi*, in North Africa. In humans, the parasite was described in 1923, by Janku, in Russia, in a child's retinal injury.

Toxoplasmosis in goats was originality mentioned by Feldman and Miller in 1956 in United States. Afterwards, Munday and Mason, (1979) described this disease as major cause of reproductive losses in this species, reporting abortion and infertility cases.

This intracellular coccidia has a predilection for the reticuloendothelial and central nervous systems. The intermediate hosts keeps the asexual phase of the cycle, transmitting the infection by ingestion of raw or undercooked meat containing *T. gondii* bradyzoite (found inside the tissue cysts, slowly multiplying, which are responsible for the cronic stage of this infection) or congenital via containing tachyzoites (stage with rapid multiplication, which is responsible for the acute phase of infection (Arias, 1994; Juránková et al., 2013).

Tachyzoites actively penetrate into intermediate hosts cells, reproducing and rapidly spreading by hematogenic via to various tissues and organs. The major clinical relevance, however, lies in placental transmission, resulting in fetal infection (Mortean, 2007). The parasitemia phase occurs approximately five days after infection and gradually decreases from two to three weeks, when the parasite cysts are formed in the tissue (Camargo, 2001).

Epidemiology

Among the animals intended for human consumption, swine, ovine and caprine are more severely infected compared with horses and cattle (Dubey and Thulliez, 1993; Lopes et al., 2013).

Among farm animals, caprine species is one of the most susceptible to *T. gondii* (Dubey and Beattie, 1988), which is more pathogenic in young animals than in adults (Dubey et al., 1985; Dubey, 1987; Dubey, 1989; Dubey, 1990; Opel et al., 1991; Pandey and Van Knapen, 1992). The positivity rate is higher in properties with presence of cats (Araujo, 1998). The hot and humid climate is favorable for the disease development, which is manifested most frequently in regions with higher rainfall and preferentially in summer months (Radostits et al., 2002). Mainly affects older animals, males and females equally, with a higher incidence in properties located close to major urban centers and with poor sanitary control (Figliuolo et al., 2004a).

The seroprevalence of *T. gondii* in small ruminants in Greece is particularly high (57.1%) (Anastasia et al., 2013). Other authors report a prevalence of 28.7% and 74% in this country (Figliuolo et al., 2004a, Figliuolo et al., 2004b, Bártová et al., 2009; Bártová et al., 2009; Panadero et al., 2010; Czopowicz et al., 2011; Hutchinson et al., 2011).

Due to its remarkable relevance to public health, epidemiological studies on toxoplasmosis in goats have been performed in Brazil. The prevalence of *T. gondii* in this country ranges from 10 to 92.4%, according to the geographical region and to the diagnostic technique utilized (Garcia et al., 2012).

Studies have record the prevalence of this disease in the world and determined a range between 3.8 and 61.3%, as demonstrated in Table 1.

In cases of pregnant goats, the protozoan invades and multiplies in the placenta and can disseminate by fetus which may cause fetal death, stillborns, birth of weak kids, or even the birth of normal animals (Pugh, 2004).

Goat products represent a risk of infection due to the high susceptibility of these animals to *T. gondii*, as exemplified by their high prevalence in the beef market, ranging up to 77% in some countries (Dubey and Beattie, 1988 Tenter et al., 2000.; EFSA, 2007; Dubey et al., 2011; Hill and Dubey, 2013; Neumayerová et al., 2014).

The isolation of this parasite was successfully performed from ovine semen (Spence et al., 1978; Lopes et al., 2009), caprine (Dubey and Sharma, 1980; Santana et al., 2010), canine (Arantes, 2005), swine (Moura et al., 2007) and cattle semen (Scarpelli et al., 2009). Santana et al. (2013), by PCR, ELISA and IFI techniques reported that, in goats, *T. gondii* infection can be sexually transmitted from male to female. The coccidia was isolated in goat tissues and their fetuses.

This is one of three pathogenic protozoan (along with *Salmonella* and *Listeria*) which represent a percentage greater than 75% of all deaths due to foodborne diseases in the U.S. (Mead et al., 1999; Dubey et al., 2011).

Table 1. Occurrence of serum antibodies against *Toxoplasma gondii* in goats from different countries

Year	Author	Local	Diagnostic technique	N°.	P	Pr (%)
1990	Vázquez et al.	Mexico	IFA	211	93	44,0
1991	Opel et al.	New Zealand	IFA	145	54	37,0
2000	Bisson et al.	Uganda	ELISA	784	240	30,6
2000	van der Puije et al.	Ghana	ELISA; IFA	526	141	26,8
2005	Jittapalapong et al.	Thailand	MAT	631	,176	27,9
2007	Sharif et al.	Iran	IFA	400	120	30,0
2008	Neto et al.	Brazil	IFA	366	112	30,6
2011	Dubey et al.	EUA	MAT	234	125	53,4
2011	Wang et al.	China	IHA	478	18	3,8
2011	Esquivel et al.	Mexico	MAT	562	174	31,0
2012	Tzanidakis et al.	Greece	ELISA	541	166	30,7
2012	Iovu et al	Romania	ELISA	662	369	55,8
2013	Anastasia et al.	EUA	ELISA	375	230	61,3
2013	Lopes et al.	Portugal	MAT	184	34	18,5

Conventions: IFA = Indirect Immunofluorescence, ELISA = Indirect immunoenzymatic assay; MAT = Modified Agglutination Test, Indirect hemagglutination (IHA).

N°. – Number of examined animals; P – Number of positive animals; Pr – Prevalence

Natural infection by *T. gondii* is mainly acquired by the ingestion of cysts found in raw or undercooked meat or through food contaminated with oocysts excreted by infected cats (Moreno et al., 2007). Subsequently, the parasite reaches the bloodstream and spreads to other tissues.

In United States, several studies have shown that 10 to 50% of the adult population has been exposed to this parasite (Dubey and Beattie, 1988, Jones et al., 2001; Jones et al., 2003; Jones et al., 2007; Dubey, 2009).

Humans can also be infected by *T. gondii* by ingestion of tachyzoites contained in goat milk and its derivatives (Millar, 2005; Dubey et al., 2011). This fact was reported by Chiari and Neves (1984) who observed the occurrence of acute toxoplasmosis in three persons of one family after ingestion of unpasteurized and not boiled goat milk. The result was confirmed by the presence of isolated tachyzoites from the goat milk, by inoculation in mice.

PATOGENY AND CLINICAL ASPECTS

The development mechanisms of lesions and clinical signs vary from mild febrile cases with lymph node enlargement, to severe cases with impairment of central nervous system, ocular abnormalities with vision loss, abortions and congenital problems (Silveira, 2001; Neves, 2003). It can also be observed acute enteritis and intestinal lesions (Dubey, 1989). Animals after 10 to 15 days of infection can manifest hyperthermia, anorexia, lethargy and weight loss during the acute phase of the disease (Santana, 2007; Fortes, 2013).

During pregnancy, premature embryonic or fetal death may occur, in addition to resorption, fetal mummification and maceration, stillborns, perinatal death or the birth of debilitated animals (Dubey, 1990; Smith and Sherman, 1994).

Pregnant goats develop nonspecific clinical feature, which can present hyperthermia, hyporexy and apathy (Chhabra et al., 1981; Dubey, 1988). The infection during the first pregnancy half may lead to major damages, although there is still a transplacental transmission risk at later stages causing less impairment of the fetus (Dubey, 1988; Vitor et al., 1991). Abortion occurs preferentially in those animals which have acquired the disease for the first time during pregnancy, approximately five to 10 days after the parasitemia stage (Radostits et al., 2002). The changes most commonly observed include: placental necrosis, encephalomyelitis, placentitis, lesions in both liver and myocardium (Dubey, 1988; Juránková et al., 2013).

Reproductive losses in a herd of goats were associated with the presence of antibodies specific to *T. gondii*. In this flock clinical signs were observed, such as pale and enlarged mesenteric lymph nodes, pneumonia with congested lung areas, encephalitis, meningoencephalitis and non-suppurative myelitis, necrotizing lymphadenitis, interstitial nephritis and periportal lymphoplasmacytic (Fialho et al., 2009). *T. gondii* is able to parasitize its host without manifesting any clinical signs, however it can lead to severe disease, especially in its congenital form (Garcia et al., 1999).

Although uncommon, death from acute disseminated toxoplasmosis has been reported in adult goats, along with encephalitis, fever, diarrhea, dyspnea, lethargy, pulmonary edema and congestion, renal infarction, multiple necrotic foci in liver and spleen, enteritis, cystitis and abomasite (Mehdi et al., 1983; Dubey, 1987). Mortality is associated with fibronecrotic lesions, congestion and edema in intestinal and pulmonary tissues, mesenteric lymph nodes infarction and focal necrosis, encephalitis, hepatitis and renal impairment, being the severity of the condition directly proportional to the amount of the inoculum (Dubey et al., 1980; Dubey, 1989; Medeiros, 2010).

DIAGNOSIS

Diagnosis is very complex and can be performed by parasitological and/or serological methods. Because this infection can assume no pathognomonic clinical features, with the great majority being asymptomatic, both in humans and in animals, the detection of antibodies by serology is essential for the diagnosis of toxoplasmosis (Figueiredo et al., 2001; Silva et al., 2002).

The diagnose of this disease can be accomplished by techniques that reveal the presence of the parasite, as bioassay (mouse inoculation), histology and immunohistochemistry, or by molecular techniques such as polymerase chain reaction (PCR), or by techniques that demonstrate the presence of antibodies against *T. gondii*, as indirect immunofluorescence reaction (IFI), Sabin-Feldman reaction, latex agglutination test (LAT), modified agglutination test (MAT), seroagglutination, indirect hemagglutination (IHA), complement fixation (CF), indirect enzyme immunoassay (ELISA) and agglutination reaction by immunoabsorption (ISAGA) (Silva et al., 2002).

In abortion cases with clinical suspicion of toxoplasmosis, it is recommended to send the placenta and fetus for laboratory diagnosis of this disease (Weissmann, 2003).

TREATMENT

Therapeutic control of toxoplasmosis is recommended only in abortion outbrakes diagnosed for the disease. In this situation, the indicated treatment includes antibiotics such as potentiated sulfonamides (trimethoprim plus sulfa), antiparasitic as decoquinate and also monensin (the latter particularly toxic and unpalatable to sheep and goats) that may be incorporated into the diet. The use of decoquinate dosed 2 mg / kg of body weight per day or addition of monensin in diet in doses varying from 15 to 30 mg / animal / day during pregnancy can significantly reduce the risk of miscarriage (Buxton et al., 1996; Radostits et al., 2002; Weissmann, 2003).

Treatment can also include the association of Sulfametazine and Pirimetamine, during three days, for three periods and in intervals of five days, reducing the toxoplasmosis effects. The drugs mentioned are efficient against the multiplying parasite, in the acute fase of the disease, although are not capable of eliminating the infection, besides having limited activity on tissue cysts forms.

CONTROL

Domestic cats (*Felis catus*) have an important role in the epidemiology of *T. gondii* by excreting oocysts in the environment thorough their feces (Dubey et al., 2004). Being these animals an increasingly present inhabitant in homes and in people's lives they deserve special attention as to their participation in the epidemiology and dissemination of this disease to farm animals in the countryside, evidencing caprines (Vidotto et al., 1990; Vargas et al., 2006). Therefore, neutering cats is important for population control (Matos et al., 2013). Rodent control is also critical in rural areas, as they are intermediate hosts in the transmission of the disease. Measures to reduce the presence of rodents include proper storage of supplies and rations, general hygiene facilities and agricultural tools. Complementing these measures, personal care and technical staff are also extremely important (Pavlovic and Ivanovic, 2005).

The fetal membranes and aborted fetuses or stillborns should be incinerated or buried in deep trenches (Dubey, 1994; Fialho et al., 2009; Fortes, 2013).

Careful exposure of pregnant and breeding females to cats, pasture, food, water and contaminated bedding are also important in the epidemiological chain of the disease (Dubey, 1994; Fortes, 2013). The control of arthropods is also essencial (flies and cockroaches) since they can act as oocysts mechanical disseminators (Pizzi, 1997).

Vaccination helps protect the flock against the clinical manifestation of the disease and persistent infections (Radostits et al., 2002).

General hygiene care, proper meat cooking and boil milk stand out as the main preventive measures of human toxoplasmosis (Jittapalapong et al., 2013; Bresciani et al., 2013; Bresciani et al., 2014).

Conclusion

Due to the importance of goat production growth in socioeconomic development, particularly for rural populations, with supply of animal protein (meat and milk), it can be stated that toxoplasmosis is an issue which causes economic losses to livestock industry, which inherent risks to public health. The animal health planning, focusing the origin of production chain, with control measures, prevention and implementation of health education programs related to awareness of producers for ways of transmission are all strategies capable to control *T. gondii* in this livestock.

References

Anastasia, D.; Elias, P.; Nikolaos, P.; Charilaos, K.; Nektarios, G. *Toxoplasma gondii* and *Neospora caninum* seroprevalence in dairy sheep and goats mixed stock farming. *Veterinary Parasitology*, 2013, vol. 198, n. 3–4, vol. 6, pp. 387–390.

Arantes, TP. Transmissão sexual do *Toxoplasma gondii* em cães (Canis familiaris). *Dissertação (Mestrado em Medicina Veterinária)* – Faculdade de Ciências Agrárias e Veterinárias, Universidade Estadual Paulista, Jaboticabal, 2005, pp. 83.

Araújo, FR.; Carvalho, CME.; Balbuena, CB. Levantamento sorológico para *Toxoplasma gondii* em bovinos de corte do Estado de Mato Grosso do Sul, Brasil. *Revista Brasileira de Medicina Veterinária*, 1998, vol.20, n.5, pp.201-203.

Arias, M.L.; Liliana, R.; Chinchilla, M.; Linder, E. Seroepidemiology of *Toxoplasma gondii* in meat producing animals in Costa Rica. *Revista de Biología Tropical*, San José, 1994, vol. 42, n.1-2, pp.15-20.

Bayat, PD.; Eslamirad, Z.; Shojaee, S. Toxoplasmosis: Experimental Vaginal Infection in NMRI Mice and Its Effect on Uterin, Placenta and Fetus Tissues. *Iranian Red Crescent Medical Journal*, 2013, vol. 15, n. 7, pp. 595–599. doi: 10.5812/ircmj.11427.

Bártová, E.; Sedlák, K.; Literák, I. *Toxoplasma gondii* and *Neospora caninum* antibodies in sheep in the Czech Republic. *Veterinary Parasitology*, 2009, vol. 161, pp. 131–132.

Bisson, A.; Maley, S.; Rubaire-Akiiki, CM.; Wastling, JM. The seroprevalence of antibodies to *Toxoplasma gondii* in domestic goats in Uganda. *Acta Tropica*, 2000, vol.76, n. 1, pp. 33–38.

Borde, G.; Lowhar, G.; Adesiyun, A. *Toxoplasma gondii* and *Chlamydophila abortus* in caprine abortions in Tobago: a sero-epidmiological study. *Journal of Veterinary Medicine B.*, 2006 vol. 53, n.4, pp. 188-194.

Bresciani, KDS.; Cardia, DFF.; Camossi, LG.; Galvão, ABG.; Vasconcellos, AL.; Santos, RR.; Santos, TR.; Soares, JA. Need for a continuing education program for toxoplasmosis control. *Education Journal*, 2013, vol. 2, n. 4, pp. 114-118.

Bresciani, KDS.; Camossi, LG.; Cardia, DFF.; Neto, LS; Matos, LVS.; Teixeira, WFP.; Soares, JA.; Santos, TR.; Gomes,JF.; Costa, AJ. Need for a continuing education program for canine toxoplasmosis control. In: Bresciani, K.D.S. Main Canine Protozoan Zoonosis. *New York: Nova Publishers*, 2014; pp. 1-14.

Buxton, D.; Path, FRC.; Whright, S.; Maley, SW.; Thomson, KM.; Millard, K. Decoquinate and the control of experimental ovine toxoplasmosis. *The Veterinary Record*, 1996, vol. 138, n.18, pp. 434-436.

Camargo, ME. Toxoplasmose. In: Ferreira, AW; Ávila, SLM. Diagnóstico Laboratorial das principais doenças infecciosas e auto-imunes, Rio de Janeiro: *Ed. Guanabara Koogan*, 2001, n.2, pp. 278-288.

Chhabra, MB.; Bhardway, RM.; Gautam, OP.; Gupta, RP. Toxoplasma infection and abortion in dairy goats. *Tropical Animal Health and Production*, 1981, vol. 13, n. 4, pp. 222-226.

Chiari, CA.; Neves, DP. Toxoplasmose humana adquirida através da ingestão de leite de cabra. *Memórias do Instituto Oswaldo Cruz*, Rio de Janeiro, 1984. vol. 79, n. 3, pp. 337-340.

Czopowicz, M.; Kabaa, J.; Szalu'-Jordanowb, O.; Nowickia, M.; Witkowskia, L.; Frymusb, T. Seroprevalence of *Toxoplasma gondii* and *Neospora caninum* infections in goats in Poland. *Veterinary Parasitology*, 2011, vol. 178, pp. 339–341.

Dubey, JP.; Sharma, SP. Prolonged excretion of *Toxoplasma gondii* in semen of goats. *American Journal of Veterinary Research*, 1980 vol. 41, pp. 794-795.

Dubey, JP. Toxoplasmosis in dogs. *Canine Practice,* 1985, Vol. 28, pp. 7-28.

Dubey, JP. Toxoplasmosis in goats. Agri-practice, New York, 1987, n.3, vol.8, pp.43-52,

Dubey, JP. Lesions in Goats Fed *Toxoplasma gondii* oocysts. *Veterinary Parasitology,* 1989, vol. 32, pp. 133-144.

Dubey, JP.; Beattie, CP. Toxoplasmosis of Animals and Humans, 1988, *CRC Press, Boca Raton*, Florida, pp. 1–220.

Dubey, JP. Status of toxoplasmosis in sheep and goats in the United States. *Journal of American Veterinary Medical Association*, 1990, vol.196, n.2.

Dubey, JP. Toxoplasmosis of Animals and Humans, CRC Press, Boca Raton, Florida, 2009, n. 2, pp. 1–313.

Dubey, J.P., Thulliez, P. Persistence of tissue cysts in edible tissues of cattle fed *Toxoplasma gondii* oocysts. *American Journal of Veterinary Research,* 1993, vol. 54, pp. 270-273.

Dubey, JP. Toxoplasmosis of Animals and Humans, 2010, *CRC Press, Boca Raton*, Florida, n. 2,

Dubey, JP. Toxoplasmosis - a waterborne zoonosis. *Veterinary Parasitology*, 2004, vol. 126, n. 1-2, pp. 57-72.

Dubey, JP.; Rajendran, C.; Ferreira, LR.; Martins, J.; Kwok, OCH.; Hill, DE.; Villena, I.; Zhou, H.; Su, C.; Jones, JL. High prevalence and genotypes of *Toxoplasma gondii* isolated from goats, from a retail meat store, destined for human consumption in the USA. *International Journal for Parasitology*, 2011, vol. 41, n. 8, pp. 827–833.

Dubey, JP. Toxoplasmosis. *Journal of American Veterinary Medical Association*, 1994, vol. 205, pp. 1593-1598.

EFSA. Monitoring of Toxoplasma in humans, food and animals. *EFSA J.*, 2007, vol. 583, pp. 1–64.

Esquivel,CA.; Aguilar, DS.; Villena,I.; Dubey, JP. Seroprevalence and correlates of *Toxoplasma gondii* infection in domestic sheep in Michoacán State, Mexico *Preventive Veterinary Medicine,* 2013, vol. 112, n. 3–4, pp. 433–437.

FAO. Food and Agriculture Organization of the United Nations. Statistical Databases. Live Animals. 2010. Disponível em:<http://faostat.fao.org /site/573/DesktopDefault.aspx?PageID=573#ancor>. Acesso em 10 de janeiro de 2014.

Feldman, H.; Miller, L. Serological study of toxoplasmosis prevalence. *American Journal of Hygiene*, 1956, vol. 64, pp. 320-335.

Fialho,CG.; Teixeira, MC.; Araujo FAP. Animal Toxoplasmosis in Brazil. *Acta Scientiae Veterinariae*, 2009 . *Acta Scientiae Veterinariae*. vol. 37, n. 1, pp. 1-23. review article Pub. 805 ISSN 1679-9216 (Online)

Figliuolo, LPC., Rodrigues, AAR, Viana, RB. Prevalence of anti-*Toxoplasma gondi* and anti-*Neospora caninum* antibodies in goat from São Paulo State, Brazil. *Small Ruminant Research*, 2004, vol. 55, pp. 29-32.a

Figliuolo, LPC.; Kasai, N.; Ragozo, AMA.; Paula, VSO.; Dias, RA.; Souza, SLP.; Gennari, SM. Prevalence of anti-*Toxoplasma gondii* and anti-*Neospora caninum* antibodies in ovine from São Paulo State, Brazil. *Veterinary Parasitology*, 2004, vol. 123, pp. 161–166.b

Figueiredo, JF.; Silva, DAO; Cabral, DD; Mineo, JR.,. Seroprevalence of *Toxoplasma gondii* in goats by the indirect haemagglutination, immunofluorescence and immunoenzymatic tests in the region of Uberlania, Brazil. *Memorias do Instituto Oswaldo Cruz*, 2001, vol. 96, n. 5, pp. 687–692.

Fortes, MS. Toxoplasmose em caprinos do estado do Paraná e comparação de testes para sorodiagnóstico. *Tese (Doutorado em Ciência Animal)* – Universidade Estadual de Londrina – 2013.

Freyre, A.; Bonino J.; Falcon, J.; Castells, D.; Correa, D.; Casaretto, A. The incidence and economic significance of ovine toxoplasmosis in Uruguay. *Veterinary Parasitology,* 1999, vol. 81, pp. 85-88.

Garcia, JL., Navarro, IT., Ogawa, L.; Oliveira, RC. Soroprevalência do *Toxoplasma gondii* em suínos, bovinos, ovinos e eqüinos e sua correlação com humanos, felinos e caninos, oriundos de propriedades rurais do norte do Paraná-Brasil. Ciência Rural, vol. 29, n.1, pp. 91-97, 1999.

Garcia, JL.; Marques, FAC.; Vidotto, O.; Navarro, IT.; Martins, GF.; Zulpo, DL.; Cunha, IAL.; Taroda, A.; Cardim, ST.; Ewald, MPC. Sero-occurrence of anti-*Toxoplasma gondii* antibodies and vertical transmission in slaughtered beef cows (*Bos indicus*). *Semina: Ciências Agrárias, Londrina*, 2012, vol. 33, n. 3, pp. 1095-1102, DOI: 10.5433/1679-0359.2012v33n3p1095

Gebremedhin,EZ.; Agonafir, A.; Tessema, TS.; Tilahun,G.; Medhin,G.; Vitale, M.; Marco, VD. Some risk factors for reproductive failures and contribution of *Toxoplasma gondii* infection in sheep and goats of Central Ethiopia: A cross-sectional study. *Research in Veterinary Science*, 2013, vol. 95, n. 3, pp. 894–900.

Hill, DE.; Dubey, JP. *Toxoplasma gondii* prevalence in farm animals in the United States. *International Journal for Parasitology*, 2013, vol. 43, n. 2, pp. 107–113 ..

Hutchinson, JP.; Wear, AR.; Lambton, SL.; Smith, RP.; Pritchard, GC. Survey to determine the seroprevalence of *Toxoplasma gondii* infection in British sheep flocks. Veterinary Record, 2011, vol. 169, pp. 582.

IBGE, 2013 <http://www.agricultura.gov.br/animal/especies/caprinos-e-ovinos>. Acesso em 25/01/2014.

Janků, J. Pathogenesis and pathologic anatomy of the "congenital coloboma" of the macula lutea in an eye of normal size, with microscopic detection of parasites in the rentna, 1923, *Cesk. Parasitology*, vol. 6, pp. 9–58.

Jittapalapong, S.; Sangvaranond, A.; Pinyopanuwat, N.; Chimnoi, W.; Khachaeram, W.; Koizumi, S.; Maruyama, S. Seroprevalence of *Toxoplasma gondii* infection in domestic goats in Satun Province, Thailand. *Veterinary Parasitology,* 2005, vol. 127, n. 1- 4, pp. 17–22.

Jones JL.; Kruszon-Moran, DK.; Wilson, M.; McQuillan, G.; Navin, T.; McAuley, JB. *Toxoplasma gondii* infection in the United States: seroprevalence and risk factors. *American Journal of Epidemiology,* 2001, vol. 154, pp. 357–65.10.1093/aje/154.4.357.

Jones, JL.; Kruszon-Moran, D.; Wilson, M. *Toxoplasma gondii* infection in the United States, 1999–2000. *Emerging Infectious Diseases journal*, 2003, vol. 9, pp. 1371–1374.

Jones, JL.; Kruszon-Moran, D; Lewis, S.; Wilson, M. *Toxoplasma gondii* infection in the United States, 1999–2004, decline from the prior decade. *The American Journal of Tropical Medicine and Hygiene*, 2007, vol. 77, pp. 405–410.

Juránková, J.; Opsteegh, M.; Neumayerová, H.; Kovařčík, K.; Frencová, A.; Baláž, V.; Volf, J.; Koudela, B. Quantification of *Toxoplasma gondii* in tissue samples of experimentally infected goats by magnetic capture and real-time PCR. *Veterinary Parasitology,* 2013, vol.193, n. 1–3, pp. 95–99.

Juránková, J.; Basso, W.; Neumayerová, H.; Baláž, V.; Jánová, E.; Sidler, X.; Deplazes, P.; Koudela, B. *Food Microbiology,* 2014, vol. 38, pp. 167–170. Brain is the predilection site of *Toxoplasma gondii* in experimentally inoculated pigs as revealed by magnetic capture and real-time PCR.

Lopes, FMR., Mitsuka-Breganó R., Gonçalves, DD.; Freire, RL.; Karigyo, CJT.; Wedy, GF.; Matsuo, T.; Reiche, EMV.; Morimoto, HK.; Capobiango, JD.; Inoue, IT.; Garcia, JL.; Navarro, IT. Factors associated with seropositivity for anti-*Toxoplasma gondii* antibodies in pregnant women of Londrina, Paraná, Brazil. *Memórias do Instituto Oswaldo Cruz,* 2009, vol.104 n. 23 pp.78-82.

Lopes, AP.; Dubey, JP.; Neto, F.; Rodrigues, A.; Martins, T.; Rodrigues, M.; Cardoso, L. Seroprevalence of *Toxoplasma gondii* infection in cattle, sheep, goats and pigs from the North of Portugal for human consumption. *Veterinary Parasitology*, 2013, vol. 193, n. 1–3, pp. 266–269.

Lovu, A.; Györke, A.; Mircean, V.; Gavrea, R.; Cozma, V. Seroprevalence of *Toxoplasma gondii* and *Neospora caninum* in dairy goats from Romania. *Veterinary Parasitology*, 2012, vol. 186, n. 3–4, pp. 470–474.

Luft, BJ.; Hafner, R.; Korzun, AH.; Leport, C.; Antoniskis, D.; Bosler, EM.; Bourland, DD.; Uttamchandani, R.; Fuhrer, J.; Jacobson, J.; Morlat, P.; Vilde, JL.; Remington, JS. Toxoplasmic encephalitis in patients with the acquired immunodeficiency syndrome. *The New England Journal of Medicine*, 1993, vol. 329, pp. 995–1000.

Matos, LVS; Teixeira, WFP.;Bregadioli, T.; Aquino, MCC.; Viol, MA. Bresciani, KDS. Orientação sobre posse responsável em uma área endêmica para Leishmaniose Visceral Canina. *Revista Ciência em Extensão*, 2012, vol.8, n.3, pp.34,

MAPA, 2014. <http://www.agricultura.gov.br/animal/especies/caprinos-e-ovinos> Acesso em 15 de janeiro de 2014.

Mead, PS.; Slutsker, L.; Dietz, V.; McCaig, LF.; Bresee, JS.; Shapiro, C.; Griffin, PM.; Tauxe, RV. Food-related illness and death in the United States. *Emerging Infectious Diseases journal*, 1999, vol. 5, pp. 607–624.

Medeiros, AD. Ocorrência da infecção por *Toxoplasma gondii* e avaliação da imunização em caprinos do Sertão do Cabugi, Rio Grande do Norte. *Dissertação de Mestrado* em Ciências Biológicas, Centro de Biociências, Universidade Federal do Rio Grande do Norte, Natal, RN. 2010, 94p.

Mehdi, NA., Kazacos, KR., Carlton, WW. Fatal disseminated toxoplasmosis in goats. *Journal of American Veterinary Medical* Association, 1983, vol. 183, n. 1, pp. 115-117.

Millar, PR. Estudo da infecção por *Toxoplasma gondii* em funcionários de um frigorífico da cidade Palmas, PR, Brasil. Revista de Patologia Tropical, 2005, vol. 3.

Montoya, JG.; Liesenfeld, O. Toxoplasmosis. *Lancet*, 2004, vol. 363, pp. 1965–1976.

Moreno, AM.; Linhares, GFC.; Sobestiansky, J.; Matos, MPC.; Barcellos, D. Doenças em Suínos. In: Sobestiansky, J. and Barcellos, D. (Eds). Goiânia: Cânone, 2007, pp. 770.

Mortean, M. C. B. et al. Diagnóstico laboratorial da infecção por *Toxoplasma gondii* na gestação. Disponível em <http://sbac.org.br/pdfs/RBAC%2039%20-%208.pdf>, 2007. Acesso em 2 de janeiro de 2014

Moura, AB.; Osaki, SC.; Zulpo, DL.; Marana, ERM. Ocorrência de anticorpos contra *Toxoplasma gondii* em suínos e ovinos abatidos no município de Guarapuava, PR, Brasil. *Revista Brasileira Parasitologia Veterinária*, 2007, *São Paulo*, vol. 16, pp. 54-56.

Munday, BL.; Mason, RW. Toxoplasmosis as a cause of perinatal death in goats. *Australian Veterinary Journal*, Artarmon, 1979. n.10, vol. 55, pp. 485-487.

Neto, JOA; Azevedo, SS; Gennari, SM; Funada, MR.; Penab, HFJ.; Araújo,ARCP.; Batista, CSA.; Silva,MLCR. Albério; Gomes, AB.; Piatti,RM.; Alves, CJ. Prevalence and risk factors for anti-*Toxoplasma gondii* antibodies in goats of the Seridó Oriental microregion, Rio Grande do Norte state, Northeast region of Brazil. *Veterinary Parasitology,* 2008, vol. 156, n. 3–4, pp. 329–332.

Neumayerová, H.; Juránková, J.; Saláková, A.; Gallas, L.; Kovařčík, K.; Koudela, B. *Food Microbiology*, 2014, vol. 39, pp. 47–52. Survival of experimentally induced *Toxoplasma gondii* tissue cysts in vacuum packed goat meat and dry fermented goat meat sausages.

Neves, DP. Parasitologia dinâmica. São Paulo: *Atheneu*, 2003, pp. 474.

Nicolle, C.; Manceaux, L. Sur une infection a` corps de Leishman (ou organismes voisins) du gondi, 1908. *Comptes Rendus Hebdomadaires des Seances de l Academie des Sciences*, vol. 147, pp. 763–766.

Opel,U.; Charleston, WAG.; Pomroy, WE.; Rommel, M. A survey of the prevalence of *Toxoplasma* infection in goats in New Zealand and a comparison of the latex agglutination and indirect fluorescence tests. *Veterinary Parasitology*, 1991, vol. 40, n. 3–4, pp. 181–186.

Panadero, R.; Painceira, A.; López, C.; Vázquez, L.; Paz, A.; Díaz, P.; Dacal, V.; Cienfuegos, S.; Fernández, G.; Lago, N.; Díez-Baños, P.; Morrondo, P. Seroprevalence of *Toxoplasma gondii* and *Neospora caninum* in wild and domestic ruminants sharing pastures in Galicia (Northwest Spain). *Research in Veterinary Science*, 2010, vol. 88, pp. 111–115.

Pandey, VS. and Van knapen, V. The seroprevalence of toxoplasmosis in sheep, goats and pigs in Zimbabwe. *Annals of Tropical Medicine and Hygiene,* 1992, vol. 86, pp. 313–315.

Pavlovic, I., Ivanovic, S. Toxoplasmosis of goats and its role and importance in pathology of goat production. *Biotechnology in Animal Husbandry*, 2005, vol. 21, n. 5-6, pp. 123-126.

Pizzi, HL. *Toxoplasmosis*. Argentina: *Rhône Poulenc Rorer,* Argentina, 1997, pp. 91.

Pugh, DG. Cliínica de ovinos e caprinos. São Paulo. *Roca*, 2004.

Radostits, OM.; Gay, CC.; Blood, DC. Doenças causadas por protozoários. In____.: *Veterinary Medicine* - A textbook of the diseases of cattle, sheep, pigs, goats and horses. Rio de Janeiro/Brasil: *Guanabara Koogan S/A*, 2002, vol. 1, n. 9, pp. 1183-1187.

Santana L.F. 2007. Toxoplasmose experimental em caprinos machos com ênfase no sistema reprodutor. 96f. Jaboticabal– SP. *Dissertação (Mestrado em Medicina Veterinária)*. Programa de Pós-Graduação em Medicina Veterinária. Universidade Estadual de São Paulo.

Santana LF.; Costa AJ.; Pieroni, J.; Lopes, WDZ.; Santos, RS.; Oliveira G.P., Mendonça R.P. and Sakamoto C.A.M. 2010. Detection of *Toxoplasma gondii* in the reproductive system of male goats. *Revista Brasileira de Parasitologia Veterinária,* 2010, vol. 19, n. 3, pp. 179-182.

Santana, LF.; Rossi, GAM.; Gaspar, RC.; Pinto, VMR.; Oliveira, GP.; Costa, AJ. Evidence of sexual transmission of *Toxoplasma gondii* in goats. *Small Ruminant Research*, 2013, vol. 115, n. 1–3, pp. 130–133.

Scarpelli, L.; Lopes WDZ.; Migani, M.; Bresciani, KDS.; Costa, AJ. *Toxoplasma gondii* in experimentally infected *Bos taurus* and *Bos indicus* semen and tissues. *Pesquisa Veterinária Brasileira*, 2009, vol. 29, pp. 59-64.

Sharif, M.; Gholami, Sh.; Ziaei, H.; Daryani, A.; Laktarashi, B.; Ziapour, SP.; Rafiei, A.; Vahedi, M. Seroprevalence of *Toxoplasma gondii* in cattle, sheep and goats slaughtered for food in Mazandaran province, Iran, during 2005. *The Veterinary Journal*, 2007, vol. 174, n. 2, pp. 422–424.

Silveira, C. Toxoplasmose - Levantamento bibliográfico de 1997-2000. *Arquivos Brasileiros de Oftalmologia,* 2001. vol. 64, pp. 263-270.

Silva, AV.; Cutolo, AA.; Langoni, H. Comparação da reação de imunofluorescência indireta e do método de aglutinação direta na detecção de anticorpos anti-toxoplasma em soros ovinos, caprinos e felinos. *Arquivos do Instituto Biológico*, 2002, vol. 69, n.1, pp. 7-11.

Skjerve, E.; Waldeland, H.; Nesbakken, T.; Kapperund, G. Risk factors for the presence of antibodies to *Toxoplasma gondii* in Norwegian slaughter lambs. *Preventive Veterinary Medicine*, 1998; vol. 35, pp. 219-227.

Smith, M.C.; Sherman, D.M. Ocular System. In____.: Goat Medicine. Ed.1. Baltimore/USA: Lippincott Williams and Wilkins, 1994, vol.1, pp.179-190.

Spence, JB.; Beattie, CP.; Faulkner, J.; Henry, L.; Watson, WA. *Toxoplasma gondii* in the semen of rams. *Veterinary Record*, 1978, vol. 14, pp. 38-39.

Tenter, AM; Heckeroth, AR; Weiss, LM. *Toxoplasma gondii*: from animals to humans. *International Journal for Parasitology*, 2000, vol. 30, pp. 1217-1258.

Tzanidakis, N.; Maksimov, P.; Conraths, FJ.; Kiossis, E.; Brozos, C.; Sotirakia, S.; Schares, G. *Toxoplasma gondii* in sheep and goats:

Seroprevalence and potential risk factors under dairy husbandry practices. *Veterinary Parasitology*, 2012, vol. 190, n. 3–4, pp. 340–348.

van der Puije, WNA.; Bosompem, KM.; Canacoo, EA.; Wastling, JM.; BD. Akanmori. The prevalence of anti-*Toxoplasma gondii* antibodies in Ghanaian sheep and goats. *Acta Tropica*, 2000, vol. 76, n. 1, pp. 21–26.

Vargas, CSG.; Cruz, MA.; Hoffman, JL.; Luz, E.; Langoni, H.; Biondo, AW. Títulos de anticorpos da classe IgG Anti-*Toxoplasma gondii* e de oocistos nas fezes de gatos de rua em Curitiba, Brasil, Anais in Conferência Sulamericana, Rio de Janeiro, 2006.

Vázquez, ZG.; Rosario-Cruz, R.; Solorzano-Salgado, M. Prevalence of antibodies against *Toxoplasma gondii* in sheep and goats in three states of Mexico. *Preventive Veterinary Medicine*, 1990, vol. 10, n. 1–2, pp. 25–29.

Vidotto O.; Navarro, IT.; Giraldi, N.; Mitsuka, R.; Freire, RL.. Estudos epidemiológicos da toxoplasmose em suínos da região de Londrina - PR. *Semina: Ciências Agrárias,* 1990, vol. 11, pp. 53-59.

Vitor, RWA; Pinto,JB.; Chiari,CA. Eliminação de *Toxoplasma gondii* através de urina, saliva e leite de caprinos experimentalmente infectados. Arquivo Brasileiro de *Medicina Veterinária e Zootecnia,* 1991, vol.43, n.2, pp. 147-154.

Wang, CR.; Qiu, JH.; Gao, JF.; Liu, LM.; Wang, C.; Liu, Q.; Yan, C.; Zhu, XQ. Seroprevalence of *Toxoplasma gondii* infection in sheep and goats in northeastern China. *Small Ruminant Research*, 2011, n. 97 , pp. 130–133.

Weissmann, J. Presumptive *Toxoplasma gondii* abortion in a sheep. *Canadian Veterinary Journal*, 2003, vol. 44, pp.322-324.

In: Recent Advances in Toxoplasmosis Research ISBN: 978-1-63117-914-3
Editor: Connor M. Lee

Chapter 5

SWINE TOXOPLASMOSIS

Juliana Ribeiro Sena Kefler[1], Maerle Oliveira Maia[1], Dulce Helena Camila dos Reis[1], Alvimar José da Costa[3], Katia Denise Saraiva Bresciani[2,3], Klaus Casaro Saturnino[1] and Thaís Rabelo dos Santos[1*]

[1]Fundação Universidade Federal de Rondônia – UNIR, Departamento de Medicina Veterinária, Campus de Rolim de Moura, Rolim de Moura, Rondônia, Brazil

[2]UNESP, Universidade Estadual Paulista Júlio de Mesquita Filho, Faculdade de Medicina Veterinária de Araçatuba, Araçatuba, São Paulo, Brazil

[3]UNESP, Universidade Estadual Paulista Júlio de Mesquita Filho, Faculdade de Ciências Agrárias e Veterinárias, UNESP, Jaboticabal, São Paulo, Brazil

ABSTRACT

Toxoplasmosis is a cosmopolitan zoonosis transmitted primarily by cats infected with the protozoan. It affects human and several other species including swine. The species merits special attention because it is considered by epidemiologists an important reservoir and source of infection to human populations due to the longevity of tissue cysts. The

[*] Corresponding author: rabelo.vet@hotmail.com.

prevalence of swine toxoplasmosis can vary greatly according to the socio-cultural habits, geographical and climatic factors. In this chapter we discuss the seroprevalence of *Toxoplasma gondii* in swines, epidemiological data, even as immunologic reactions of organic animal front ace infections, the main forms of diagnosis used and the possible advances that can contribute to the prevention of these animals.

INTRODUCTION

Toxoplasma gondii was first described in South Africa by Nicolle & Manceaux (1908), in a rodent (*Ctenodactylus gundi*), but only in 1909 they confirmed as a new protozoan. In Brazil, Splendore in 1908 isolated in a laboratory in São Paulo this parasite into a rabbit. However, only in the early 70's that was reported coccidial its nature as well as their definitive hosts of *Toxoplasma gondii* and intermediate (Frenkel et al., 1970). The felines are the definitive hosts (Motta et al., 2008), with that domestic cats play an important role in disease transmission to all humans and warm-blooded animals (Garcia, 2006).

Toxoplasmosis is a parasitic disease that occurs worldwide (Dubey & Beattie, 1988; Dubey, 2009). Therefore brings huge economic losses to livestock and comes harming public health, as a zoonosis. *T. gondii* is an obligate intracellular protozoan of life (Silva, 2003). Belonging to the phylum Apicomplexa, order Eucoccidiila, Sarcocystidae family, genus toxoplasma (Fialho, et al., 2009) Toxoplasma signifies an arch in which toxon: arc and plasma: form (Neves, 2009).

The life cycle of *T. gondii* occurs in two forms: as sexual (enteroepitelial cycle) and asexual (extra intestinal cycle) (Dubey, 2010). During its development, the *T. gondii* goes through three distinct stages: tachyzoites, bradyzoites and sporozoites (Dubey, 2008). Tachyzoites is found in the acute phase of the disease. These may be free within the organic or parasitological vacuoles of phagocytic cells of the monocytic system liquid.

The bradyzoites can also be referred in tissues during chronic phase (Kawazoe, 2005). And sporozoites, oocysts, which is present in the feces of cats has not immune and double membrane which confers resistance to the parasite (Dubey & Beattie 1988), the deleted sporulate oocyst within three days, and may remain for up to two years in ambient conditions in viable (Neves, 2009).

SWINE TOXOPLASMOSIS

T. gondii infection in pigs was first diagnosed by Farrell et al. (1952) in the United States of America in the herd had increased mortality in all age groups (Mylar, 2008). In Brazil, the swine toxoplasmosis was first described by Silva (1959) in the State of Minas Gerais, in pigs at 28 days after birth in which this protozoan found in the lungs, heart, liver and mesenteric lymph nodes.

Swine become infected from ingestion of oocysts, which is released by cat feces and can contaminate the food came, soil, water, food scraps and other transmission form is vertical (Dubey et al., 1995; Wang, et al. 2002). Toxoplasmosis has a higher prevalence of this animal. The pigs at slaughter are not tested for *T. gondii* infection, why not meat inspections allow the detection of cysts that has a size of 100 lm generally (Basso et al., 2013).

Humans can be infected came from ingestion of tissue cysts in pigs (Tender et al., 2000 Kijlstra & Jongert, 2008) that can survive more than two years, being one of the most common source of infection is the consumption of raw or undercooked meat (Dubey et al., 1991, 1998; Garcia, 2009), and ingestion of food and water with sporulated oocyst (Dubey & Jones, 2008). Immunocompromised individuals and pregnant women are more susceptible to this infection (Pozio, 2004; Alvarado-Esquivel, et al., 2009.).

The prevalence of *T. gondii* infection in swine is influenced by husbandry conditions and may vary from 0% to over 90% (Pardini et al., 2012), thus being influenced by management system (Dubey, 2009a). Pigs reared outdoors may have infection rates of approximately 50-90% (Gebreyes et al., 2008).

In Europe, in the mid 90 the pigs were raised in the intensive management system, in which the prevalence has been declining gradually for example, in Austria, the seroprevalence was 14% in ten years in 1982 became 0.9% (Edelhofer, 1994; Dubey, 2009a). Currently on the European continent is emerging a new fad that is the creation of outdoor pigs, i.e., organic animals, this trend may increase the prevalence in pigs in the Netherlands (Meerburg, et al., 2006; Kijstra, et al., 2008).

In the United States in a period of 20 years was observed that animals of containment before recorded prevalence from 23% currently to be 2.7% (Dubey et al., 1991; Dubey, 2009b; Hill et al., 2010.). China pig meat is the most consumed having a toxoplasmosis seroprevalence of 24.5% (Tao et al., 2011), in Brazil is reported of 43, 7% (Calvacante et al., 2006).

According Prickett et al. (1985), means a pig which has had an infection by *T. gondii* has 85% chance of having viable agent in your body. The prevalence of swine toxoplasmosis may vary from region to region, as the socio-cultural, geographic and climatic factors found habits. Toxoplasmosis in swine is a matter of food safety (Wang, et al., 2002).

In accordance with Moura et al. (2007) and Bezerra et al. (2009) the occurrence of the disease in swine is more frequent in females than in males. This behavior, however, is probably due more to a sampling bias than a sex-linked susceptibility. However, the influence of *T. gondii* pig is clearly age-dependent (Wang, et al. 2002).

Another relevant factor pointed out by Silva et al. (2008), is the age of the animal. This being important in assessing the risk of infection by the consumption of pork meat and its derivatives. In general, the fresh beef is from animals younger age, while the inlays are often produced by animal disposal, usually older and, according to the literature, most commonly infected.

Pathogenesis and Clinical Signs

In swine, infection with *T. gondii* carries reproductive disorder, death, mummification and embryo reabsorption, abortion (Dubey, 2004) and clinical disorders such as anorexia, prostration, hyperthermia, dyspnea, weakness of the posterior members nasal discharge, fever, cyanosis and death (Bezerra et al., 2009; Dubey, 2009).

Exposure of women to *T. gondii* during the first third of pregnancy may result in prenatal death or serious birth defects. The infection in immunocompromised humans, for example, cancer, AIDS, transplant can result in encephalitis, and blindness (Navarro et al. 1992).

Diagnosis

The diagnosis is very important because of the disease is a zoonosis and manifests itself in different ways and situations with clinical signs that can be easily confused with other infectious diseases such as viral infections, leptospirosis, brucellosis, chlamydiosis and neosporosis, these infections also spread among domestic animals (Neves, 2005). Laboratory testing of *T. gondii* in pigs may be performed through two direct and indirect methods.

Direct methods, demonstration of coccidia, examination of infected tissues however the sensitivity is limited because of the sample size, and low parasite load (Dubey, 2009). However, are always used during the acute phase of the disease, because it is easier to find tachyzoites in blood, cerebrospinal fluid, saliva, milk, placenta than locating a hidden cyst in some organ of the patient is in the chronic phase (Neves, 2009).

The indirect methods should be performed from the use of immunological diagnosis, the presence of specific antibodies by serology. Several other immunological methods have been used as indirect hemagglutination (IHA), the modified agglutination test (MAT) (Dubey, 1997), polymerase chain reaction (PCR) detection of genetic material, indirect immunofluorescence assay (IFA), enzyme immunoassay (ELISA) (Costa et al. 2007), the latter two are capable of detecting IgM and IgG, then it is a pattern (Neves, 2009).

According to Dubey et al. (1997) The MAT test is a highly sensitive for use in pigs with high analytical specificity, being less sensitive than the ELISA only. In accordance with Araújo (1999) Use of IFAT for the diagnosis, investigations and epidemiological surveys have been universally accepted, both for humans and other animal species, it is considered easy to perform and highly sensitive. Have the results of Minho et al. (2004) are interesting because no differences between IFA and MAT. Therefore, the combination of two or more methods of analysis reveals the actual infection and aids in the same stage of differentiation (Kompalic et al. 2004).

Pathology and Immunology

Pathological and immunological changes occur in *T. gondii* infection in swine, with that many researchers have been devoted to study these transformations. Vidotto et al. (1987) demonstrated that in pigs inoculated oocyst of AS28 strains between days 42-50 of gestation abortion occurred. In addition, these animals showed tachypnea, nasal discharge, prostration, neutropenia, lymphocytes, monocytes, eosinopenia. Have nuts with 70-93 days of gestation was recorded fetal mummification. In pathological examinations of nuts congestive and hemorrhagic lesions of the central nervous system, liver, lungs, spleen, kidney, skeletal muscle and final portion of the small intestine were found. In addition to the fetus and suckling except said small intestine injury were no lesions in the large intestine.

Silva et al. (1994) studied the immunogenicity and antigenicity of five samples from *T. gondii* when inoculated intravenously into pig and found that the surface antigens are common to several samples tested role in the response to the immunodominant antibody production.

In Londrina/PR, Giraldi et al. (1996) cases of congenital toxoplasmosis were detected in a swine farms. From a total of 43 matrices associated with reproductive disorders, 24 (55.81%) were positive for anti-T serum antibodies. gondii. In five cases parasitemia was detected, and in 12 cases the mice inoculated with samples from aborted or stillborn animals had antibodies against the parasite. Immunohistochemistry was positive in 12 of 20 cases examined, marked tachyzoites and tissue cysts in samples of brain, spleen, liver, retina, muscles and lungs.

Nishi (2004) investigated the expression of genes associated with immune response in pigs inoculated orally with oocysts of the strain VEG response and discovered that pigs showed an initial response related to innate mechanisms of acute inflammation and the immune response beginning at two days post - infection, peaking at four and seven and a decrease at 14 days.

In five pigs infected orally with 5000 oocysts of *T. gondii* strains M7741 Silva (2009) found that at 30 days post-infection increased from 4.2% in the thickness of the wall of the jejunum, 9.7% at the time villi and 23.9% in the muscular wall. 60 DPI changes intensified, with a 25.1% increase in the total wall, 18.6% in the muscular wall, 32.0% in the tunica mucosa and 12.8% in villous height. In these same animals, neuronal death was not found, but hypertrophy of neurons can therefore be concluded that infection with *T. gondii* resulted in increased contractility of the intestine and is a response of the body to eliminate the infection, evidenced mainly by the occurrence of diarrhea in experimentally infected animals throughout the experiment.

Prevention and Control

According to Farias, (2002) knowledge of effective forms of human and animal infection with *Toxoplasma gondii* and the biological and epidemiological characteristics of the parasite is crucial for physicians and veterinarians recommend effective measures to control the disease.

Despite the absence a standard way of controlling or preventing that is globally effective due to the versatility of the *T. gondii* and its complex epidemiology, general care that will serve as a control for most locations should be taken (Tenter et al., 2000). One way to prevent infection is to inactivate the cysts in meat of animals by brining (Navarro et al., 1992.), heating (Neto & Marchi, 1999) and freezing (Remington & Desmonts, 1995; Kijlstra & Jongert, 2009).

Other measures to prevent human infection is to wash your hands thoroughly after handling raw meat with, vegetables, and after contact with the earth (Fialho et al., 2009) and this further recommendation immunocompromised persons or pregnant women.

Prevention of cats is needed that is not offered raw or undercooked meat, viscera or live animals, and avoid leaving the house, avoiding the hunting and offer only commercial feed (Neves, 2003). The cat has an important role in the transmission of toxoplasmosis, the presence of this animal in the swine farms should be avoided (Vidotto, et al., 1990, Dubey, 1998).

Conclusion

Toxoplasmosis in swine has much still to be investigated particularly in respect say about the control of rodents, cats that come into contact with these animals in confinement, either in their food or in their water troughs, simple measures can be avoided. Another situation that has been gaining attention is the new trend of organic swinein which research had shown that a significant increase in the seroprevalence of toxoplasmosis in swine compared those who are raised in confinement system. There must be standardized in the processing of meat, such as suitable temperature, curing conditions, curing lead to the death of the oocysts that is in tissue. Therefore, it is is extremely important that new studies are performed in swine toxoplasmosis.

References

Alvarado-Esquivel, C; Torres-Castonera, A; Liesenfeld, O; García-López, CR; Estrada-Martínez, A; Sifuentes-Álvarez, A; Marsal-Hernández, JF; Esquivel-Cruz, R; Sandoval-Herrera, F; Castaneda, JA; Dubey, J. Seroepidemiology of *Toxoplasma gondii* infection in pregnant woman in rural Durango, México. *J. Parasitol.*, v. 95, 271–274, 2009.

Araujo, FAP. de Avaliação soroepidemiológica de anticorpos para *Toxoplasma gondii* Nicolle & Manceaux, 1909 em soros de suínos (*Sus scrofa*) da região da Grande Erechim, RS – Brasil, detectados através das técnicas de imunofluorescência indireta de imunoenzimática. 1999. 125f. Tese (Doutorado na área de Protozoologia) - Instituto Oswaldo Cruz.

Basso, W; Hartnack, S; Pardini, L; Maksimov, P; Koudela, B; Venturini, MC; Schares, G; Sidler, X; Lewis, FI; Deplazes, P. Assessment of diagnostic accuracy of a commercial ELISA for the detection of *Toxoplasma gondii* infection in pigs compared with IFAT, TgSAG1-ELISA and Western blot, using a Bayesian latent class approach. *International Journal for Parasitology*, v.43, 565-570, 2013.

Bezerra, RA; Paranhos, EB; Del'arco, AE; Albuquerque, GR. 2009. Detection anti-*Toxoplasma gondii* antibodies in swines bred and abated in the Bahia State, Brazil. *Rev. Bras. Parasitol. Vet*, Jaboticabal, v. 18, n. 3, 78-80.

Cavalcante, GT; Aguiar, DM; Chiebao, D; Dubey, JP; Ruiz, VLA; Dias, RA; Camargo, LMA; Labruna, MB; Gennari, SM. Seroprevalence of *Toxoplasma gondii* antibodies in cats and pigs from rural western Amazon, *Brasil. J. Parasitol*, v. 92, 863–864, 2006.

Costa, TL; Silva, MG; Rodrigues, IMX; Barbaresco, AA; Avelino, MM; Castro, AM. Diagnóstico clínico e laboratorial da toxoplasmose. *Newsla*, v. 85, 88-104, 2007.

Dias, RAF; Freire, RL. Surtos de toxoplasmose em seres humanos e animais. *Semina, Ciênc. Agrárias*, Curitiba, v. 26, n. 2, 239-247, 2005.

Dubey, JP. Validation of the specificity of the modified agglutination test for toxoplasmosis in pigs. *Vet. Parasitol*, v.71, 307-10, 1997.

Dubey, JP. Advances in the life cicle of *Toxoplasma gondii*. *Int. J. Parasitol*, v. 28, 1019-1024, 1998.

Dubey, JP. Toxoplasmosis in pigs- The last 20 years. *Vet. Parasitol*, v. 164, 89-103, 2009a.

Dubey, JP. Toxoplasmosis of Animals and Humans. *2nd ed. CRC Press, Boca Raton, Florida, in press.* 2009b.

Dubey, JP. Toxoplasmosis of Animals and Humans, *2nd ed. CRC Press, Boca Raton*, 313, 2010.

Dubey, JP; Murrel, KD; Fayer, R. Persistence of encysted *T. gondii* in tissues of pigs fed oocysts. *American J. of Vet. Research*, v.45, 941-1943, 1984.

Dubey, JP; Towle, A. Toxoplasmosis in sheep. St Albans, UK, *Commonwealth Institute of Parasitology*, 11, 1986.

Dubey, JP; Beattie, CP. Toxoplasmosis of Animals and Man. *CRC Press, Boca Raton, FL*, 220, 1988.

Dubey, JP; Urban, JF; Davis, SW. Protective immunity to toxoplasmosis in pigs vaccinated with nonpersistent strain of *Toxoplasma gondii*. *American J. of Vet. Research*, v. 52, 1316–1319, 1991.

Dubey, JP; Baker, DG; Davis, SW; Urban, JF; Shen, SK. Persistence of immunity to toxoplasmosis in pigs vaccinated with a non persistent strain of *Toxoplasma gondii. American J. of Vet. Research*, v. 55, n.7, 982-987, 1994.

Dubey, JP; Weigel, RM; Siegel, AM; Thulliez, P; Kitron, UD; Mitchell, MA; Mannelli, A; Mateus-Pinilla, NE; Shen, SK; Kwok, OCH; Todd, KS. Sources and reservoir of *Toxoplasma gondii* infection on 47 swine farms in Illinois. *J. Parasitol*, v. 81, 723–729, 1995.

Dubey, JP; Thulliez, P; Powell, EC. *Toxoplasma gondii* in Iowa sows: comparison of antibody titers to isolation of *T. gondii* by bioassays in mice and cats. *J. Parasitol*, v.81, n.1, 48-53, 1995.

Dubey, JP; Navarro, IT; Sreekumar, C; Dahl, E; Freire, RL; Kawabata, HH; Vianna, MCB; Kwok, OCH; Shen, SK; Thulliez, P; Lehmann, T. *Toxoplasma gondii* infections in cats from Parana´, Brazil: seroprevalence, tissue distribution, and biologic and genetic characterizations of isolates. *J. Parasitol*, v. 90, 721–726, 2004.

Dubey, JP; Hill, DE; Sundar, N; Velmurugan, GV; Bandini, LA; Kwok, OCH; Pierce, V; Kelly, K; Dulin, M; Thulliez, P; Iwueke, C; Su, C. Endemic toxoplasmosis in pigs on a farm in Maryland: isolation and genetic characterization of *Toxoplasma gondii*. *J. Parasitol*, v. 94, 36–41, 2008.

Dubey, JP; Jones, JL. *Toxoplasma gondii* infection in humans and animals in the United States. *Int. J. Parasitol*, v. 38, 1257–1278, 2008.

Edelhofer, R. Prevalence of antibodies against *Toxoplasma gondii* in pigs in Austria—an evaluation of data from 1982 and 1992. *Parasitol. Res.*, v. 80, 642–644, 1994.

Faria, IG; Ferreira, JM; Garcia, SK. Mercado consumidor de carne suína e derivada em Belo Horizonte. *Arq. Bras. Med. Vet. Zootec.*, v. 58, 251-6, 2006.

Farrel, RL; Docton, FL; Chamberlain, DM; et al. Toxo-6. plasmosis. 1. Toxoplasma isolated from swine. *Am. J. Vet. Res.*, v. 13, 181-5, 1952.

Fialho, CG; Teixeira, MC; De Araujo, FAP. Toxoplasmose animal no Brasil. *Acta Scientiae Veterinariae*, v. 37, n. 1, 1-23, 2009.

Frenkel, JK; Dubey, JP; Miller, NL. *Toxoplasma gondii* in cats: fecal stage identified as coccidia oocists. *Science*, v.167, 893-896, 1970.

Garcia, JL; Navarro, IT; Vidotto, O; Genneari, SM; Machado, RZ; Pereira, ABL; Sinhorini, IL. *Toxoplasma gondii*: Comparison of a rhoptry-ELISA in sera of experimentally intected pigs. *Experimental Parasitology*, v. 113, 100-105, 2006.

Garcia, JL. Vaccination concepts against *Toxoplasma gondii. Exp. Rev. Vaccines*, v. 6, 215–225, 2009.

Gebreyes, WA; Bahnson, PB; Funk, JA; Mckean, J; Patchanee, P. Seroprevalence of *Trichinella, Toxoplasma, and Salmonella* in antimicrobial- free and conventional swine production systems. *Foodborne Pathog. Dis.*, v. 5, 199–203, 2008.

Giraldi, N; Freire, RL; Navarro, IT. Toxoplasmose congênita natural em granjas de suínos em Londrina, PR. *Arq. Bras. Med. Vet. Zoot.*, v. 48, 83-90, 1996.

Hill, DE; Haley, C; Wagner, B; Gamble, HR; Dubey, JP. Seroprevalence of and risk factors for *Toxoplasma gondii* in the US swine herd using sera collected during the National Animal Health Monitoring Survey (Swine 2006). *Zoonoses Public Health*, v. 57, 53-59, 2010.

Kawazoe, U. *Toxoplasma gondii.* In: Neves D.P. (Ed.) *Parasitologia Humana.* 11.ed. São Paulo: Atheneu, 494, 2005.

Kijlstra, A; Jongert, E. Control of the risk of human toxoplasmosis transmitted by meat. *Int. J. Parasitol*, v. 38, 1359–1370, 2008.

Kijlstra, A; Meerburg, B; Cornelissen, J; De Craeye, S; Vereijken, P; Jongert, E. The role of rodents and shrews in the transmission of *Toxoplasma gondii* to pigs. *Vet. Parasitol*, v. 156, 183–190, 2008.

Kijlstra, A; Jongert, E. Toxoplasma-safe meat: close to reality? *Trends Parasitol*, v. 25, n. 1, 18–22, 2009.

Kompalic-Cristo, A; Nogueira, SA; Guedes, AL. Lack of technical specificity in the molecular diagnosis of toxoplasmosis. *Trans. R. Soc. Trop. Med. Hyg.*, v. 98, 92-5, 2004.

Koski, VH. Evaluation of ELISA for the Dectction of Toxoplasma Antibodies in Swine Sera. *Acta vet. Scand.*, v. 31, 413-422, 1990.

Meerburg, BG; Van Riel, JW; Cornelissen, JB; Kijlstra, A; Mul, MF. Cats and goat whey associated with *Toxoplasma gondii* infection in pigs. *Vector-Borne Zoonotic Dis.*, v. 6, 266–274, 2006.

Milar, PR; Sobreiro, LG; Bonna, ICF; Amendoeira, MRR. The importance of food animals in the infection for *Toxoplasma gondii* in Brazil. *Ciências Agrárias, Londrina*, v. 29, n. 3, 693-706, 2008.

Minho, AP; Freire, RL; Vidotto, O. Evaluation of the indirect fluorescent antibody test and modified agglutination test for detection of antibodies against *Toxoplasma gondii* in experimentally infected pigs. *Pesq Vet Bras*, v. 24, 199-202, 2004.

Motta, ACDA; Vieira, MIB; Bondan, C; Edelweiss, MIA; Dametto, MA; Gomes, A. Aborto em ovinos associados à toxoplasmose: caracterização sorológica, anátomo- patológica e imunohistoquímica. *Rev. Bras. Parasitol. Vet*, v. 17, n. 1, 204-208, 2008.

Moura, AB; Osaki, SC; Zulpo, DL. Ocorrência de anticorpos contra *Toxoplasma gondii* em suínos e ovinos abatidos no município de Guarapuava, PR, Brasil. *Rev. Bras. Parasitol, Vet.*, v. 16, 54-6, 2007.

Navarro, IT; Vidotto, O; Giraldi, N; Freire, RL. *Toxoplasma gondii*: Isolamento a partir de carne e cérebro de suínos comercializados na região de Londrina, *Semina*, v.13, 5-18, 1992.

Neto, VA; Marchi, CR. Toxoplasmose. In: Cimerman B. & Cimerman S. (Eds). *Parasitologia Humana e seus Fundamentos Gerais. São Paulo: Atheneu*, 375, 1999.

Neves, DP. Parasitologia humana. *11ª. Ed. São Paulo, Atheneu*, p. 494, 2005.

Neves, DP. Parasitologia dinâmica. *03ª. Ed. São Paulo, Atheneu*, p. 592, 2009.

Nicolle, C; Manceaux, L. Sur une infection à corps de Leishman (ou organisms voisins) du gondii. *C. R. Herbd Séances Acad. Sci.*, v. 147, 763- 766, 1908.

Nishi, SM. Efeito da infecção pelo *Toxoplasma gondii* na expressão de genes associados à resposta imune em tecidos de suínos [tese]. São Paulo (SP): Universidade de São Paulo; 2004.

Pardini, L; Maksimov, P; Herrmann, DC; Bacigalupe, D; Rambeaud, M; Machuca, M; Moré, G; Basso, W; Schares, G; Venturini, MC. Evaluation of an in-house TgSAG1 (P30) IgG ELISA for diagnosis of naturally acquired *Toxoplasma gondii* infection in pigs. *Veterinary Parasitology*, v. 189, 2004-210, 2012.

Pozio, E. Highly active antiretroviral therapy and opportunistic protozoan infections. *Parassitologia*, v. 46, 89–93, 2004.

Prickett, MD; Dreesen, DW; Waltman, WD; Blue, JL; Brown, J. Correlation of tissue infection and findings in pigs fed *Toxoplasma gondii* oocysts. *Am. J. Vet. Res.*, v.46, n. 5, 1130-1132, 1985.

Remington, JS; Mcleod, R; Desmonts, G. Toxoplasmosis. In: Remington, J.S., Klein, J.O. (Eds.), Infectious Diseases of the Fetus & Newborn Infant, *4th Edition. Saunders, Philadelphia*, 140–268,1995.

Silva, IML. Sobre um caso de toxoplasmose espontânea em suínos. *Arq. Esc. Super. Vet. Univ. Rural. Est. Minas Gerais*, v. 12, 425-8, 1059.

Silva, DS; Bahia-Oliveira, LMG; Shen, SK; Kwok, OCH; Lehman, T; Dubey, JP. Prevalence of *Toxoplasma gondii* in chickens from a area in southern Brazil Highly Endemic to Humans. *Journal of Parasitology*, Lawrence, v. 89, n. 2, 394-396, 2003.

Silva, ACB; Mitsuka, R; Navarro, IT. Avaliação pela imunofluorescência indireta dos aspectos imunogênicos e antigênicos de diferentes amostras de *Toxoplasma gondii* inoculadas em suínos. *Rev. Bras. Parasitol. Vet.*, v. 3, 17-22, 1994.

Silva, AV; Boareto, H; Isbrecht, FB. Ocorrência de anticorpos anti-*Toxoplasma gondii* em suínos da região oeste do Paraná, Brasil. *Vet Zootec.* v. 15, 263-6, 2008.

Silva, PC. Análise morfométrica da parede e dinâmica do epitélio do jejuno de suínos com toxoplasmose [dissertação]. Umuarama (PR): Universidade Paranaense; 2009.

Tao, Q; Wang, Z; Feng, H; Fang, R; Nie, H; Hu, M; Zhou, Y; Zhao, J. Seroprevalence and risk factors of *Toxoplasma gondii* infection in pig farms in central China. *J. Parasitol*, v. 97, 262–264, 2011.

Tenter, AM; Heckeroth, AR; Weiss, LM. Toxoplasma gondii: from animals to humans. *Int. J. Parasitol.*, v. 30, 1217–1258, 2000.

Vidotto, O; Costa, AJ. Toxoplasmose experimental em porcas gestantes. II. Parasitemia e resposta imunitária humoral. *Arq. Bras. Med. Vet. Zoot.*, v. 39, 783-94, 1987.

Vidotto, O; Costa, AJ. Toxoplasmose experimental em porcas gestantes. III. Alterações patológicas e reisolamento. *Arq. Bras. Med. Vet. Zoot.*, v. 39, 795-814, 1987.

Vidotto, O; Navarro, IT; Giraldi, N; Freire, RL; Mitsuka, R. Estudos epidemiológicos da toxoplasmose em suínos da região de Londrina, *Semina*, v.11, 53–59, 1990.

Wang, CH; Diderrich, V; Kliebenstein, K; Patton, S; Zimmerman, J; Hallam, A; Bush, E; Faulkner, C; Mccord, R. *Toxoplasma gondii* levels in swine operations: differences due to technology choice and impact on costs of production. *Food Control*, v. 13, 103-106, 2002.

In: Recent Advances in Toxoplasmosis Research ISBN: 978-1-63117-914-3
Editor: Connor M. Lee

Chapter 6

RECENT ADVANCES IN OVINE TOXOPLASMOSIS AND PUBLIC HEALTH ASPECTS

Lucilene Granuzzio Camossi[1,*], Daniel Fontana Ferreira Cardia[2], Helio Langoni[1], Thais Rabelo dos Santos[3], Lucas Vinicius Shigaki de Matos[4], Julia Cestari Pierucci[4], Jancarlo Ferreira Gomes[5], Alexandre Xavier Falcão[5], Alvimar José da Costa[4] and Katia Denise Saraiva Brescani[2,4]

[1]UNESP, Universidade Estadual Paulista Júlio de Mesquita Filho, Faculdade de Medicina Veterinária e Zootecnia de Botucatu, Botucatu, São Paulo, Brazil
[2]UNESP, Universidade Estadual Paulista Júlio de Mesquita Filho, Faculdade de Medicina Veterinária de Araçatuba, Araçatuba, São Paulo, Brazil
[3]UNIR, Fundação Universidade Federal de Rondônia, Departamento de Medicina Veterinária, Campus de Rolim de Moura, Rolim de Moura, Rondônia, Brazil
[4]UNESP, Universidade Estadual Paulista Júlio de Mesquita Filho, Faculdade de Ciências Agrárias e Veterinárias, Jaboticabal, São Paulo,Brazil

[*] E-mail: lucilenecamossi@gmail.com.

[5]UNICAMP, Universidade de Campinas,
Instituto de Biologia e Computação, Campinas, São Paulo, Brazil

Abstract

Toxoplamosis is considered major parasitary disease in sheep, due its importance in veterinary medicine and animal science and in public health. In ewe the main clinical repercussion is abortion, economic losses through embryonic and fetal death, still birth and neonatal losses, represents an obstacle in profitability in worldwide sheep farm production. Amongst food producing animals, sheep meat was considered to be highest risk food for transmission of toxoplasmosis to humans, furthermore recent studies have been found cases of excretion of the parasite from milk of naturally infected sheep, suggesting a potential source of infection to humans when consumed without prior boiling or pasteurization, which can facilitate the zoonotic transmission. New research has shown that repeat ovine transmission of *T. gondii* in subsequent pregnancies can occur, unlike previous studies suggest that sheep have aborted due to parasite develop protection against future abortion. In these animals is likely that reactivation of latent toxoplasmosis can occur and influence the high incidence of infection in sheep. The main objective of this chapter will be discussing important aspects involving new advances in the epidemiology, diagnosis and control of this important disease in sheep industry.

Introduction

The protozoan parasite *Toxoplasma gondii*, belonging to the apicomplexan phylum, is one of the most successful parasites worldwide and is able to infect all warm blooded animals including people (Gangneux and Dardé, 2012), it is considered major parasitary disease in ovine, due its importance in veterinary medicine and animal science and in public health (Bresciani et al., 2013).

The according to Veterinary Investigation Diagnosis Analysis (2009) toxoplasmosis was considered the second most commonly diagnosed disease of abortion in sheep, after Chlamydiosis. Sheep are more susceptible to *T. gondii* infection compared to others livestock animals and the main clinical repercussion is abortion, economic losses through embryonic and fetal death, still birth and neonatal losses, represents an obstacle in profitability in worldwide sheep farm production (Buxton et al., 2007; Dubey, 2009; Cenci Goga et al., 2011; Edwards and Dubey, 2013).

EPIDEMIOLOGY

Serological studies show the presence of this parasite in sheep in different continents and their global importance, which may represent a good marker of the potential risk for human infections (Gebremedhin et al., 2013). In Africa, seroprevalence of *T. gondii* antibodies in sheep was 31,59% in Ethiopia (Gebremedhin et al., 2013), 71% in Libya (Al-Mabruk et al., 2013). The Americas were reported prevalence of 94,8% in USA (Edward and Dubey, 2013), 22,1% in Brazil (Andrade et al., 2013), 17,3% in Argentina (Hecker et al., 2013) and 23,1% in Mexico (Alvarado-Esquivel et al., 2013). On the European continent seroprevalences was 33,6% in Portugal (Lopes et al., 2013), 33,97% in Italy (Sechi et al., 2013), 36% in Ireland (Halová et al., 2013) and 49,3% in Spain (García-Bocanegra et al., 2013). In Asia, the prevalence was 4,4% in China (Yang et al., 2013), 3,4% in Iran (Heidari et al., 2013). In sheep from New Zealand, prevalence was 85% (Dempster et al., 2011).

Previously toxoplasmosis has been associated with pork meat, but with the intensive management pig production, which places barriers to infection from the environment and cats, this has led to a marked drop in the *T. gondii* seroprevalence in pork (Dubey et al., 2005; Gangneux and Dardé 2013). Currently, amongst food producing animals, sheep meat was considered to be highest risk food for transmission of toxoplasmosis to humans, infected animals can contain a large numbers of bradyzoites containing tissue cysts in their meat, in many different tissues, mainly in the muscles and brain (Dubey and Jones, 2008). Studies indicate that viable *T. gondii* parasites have been recovered from as many as 67% of sheep tissue samples (Gangneux and Dardé 2013) and although toxoplasmosis is emphatically associated with felines, its definitive hosts, currently it is estimated that 50% of cases are foodborne (Scallan et al., 2011). Therefore, *T. gondii* were classified as high priority for sheep meat inspection by the European Food Safety Authority (2013), due high public health relevance based on their high severity and on the evidence of meat as a risk factor for human zoonotic transmission.

Furthermore recent studies have been found cases of excretion of the parasite from milk of naturally infected sheep, suggesting a potential source of infection to humans when consumed without prior boiling or pasteurization, which can facilitate the zoonotic transmission, it was a relevant result for public health since milk and dairy products are important food sources in rural areas, where milk is used for subsistence without pasteurization or boiling prior to consumption (Fusco et al., 2007; Camossi et al., 2011).

The presence of cats on the pasture farm has always been considered an important risk factor for acquisition of infection due to a greater environmental contamination of pastures with oocysts eliminated in the feces of felids, definitive host of toxoplasmosis, an infected cat may shed millions of oocysts into the environment and it only requires 20 oocysts to cause infection and disease in naïve sheep (McColgan et al., 1988). Same importance should be given to drinking water which has also been considered as an important means of agent transmission, both sources of still water our running water, acting as a disseminator of oocysts in flocks of sheep (Andrade et al., 2013), recent studies indicate that contaminated water may be as important, if not more important a source of infection than contaminated feed (Cenci-Goga et al., 2013; Andrade et al., 2013).

In public health, according to methods to estimate disease impact such as Disability Adjusted Life Years (DALYS) has shown that toxoplasmosis to be one of the most significant food borne pathogens across the world (Kortbeek et al., 2009). In sheep industry, represents a threat for consumers, who can be infected by raw or undercooked meat and untreated milk, with consequences at high risk for severe toxoplasmosis mostly for pregnant women and immunologically compromised individuals, as in HIV infected (Innes et al., 2009; Dubey et al, 2009; Cenci-Goga et al., 2011). Currently, toxoplasmosis has been reported more frequently also in healthy individuals, this is most common infectious etiology of posterior uveitis in immunocompetent persons (Bonfioli and Orefice, 2005). It is now recognized that the genotype of the strain of *T. gondii*, may influence clinical severity, atypical strains were linked severe clinical manifestations even in immunocompetent individuals (Gangneux and Dardé, 2012).

Patogeny and Clinical Signs

The severity of congenital infection vary the stage of pregnancy at which sheep becomes infected, infection during the early stage of gestation can result in fetal death, resorption, and abortion, however if infection occurs in the latter stage of gestation, the effects are less severe or may have no clinical effect and lambs are usually born normal, but infected and immune (Buxton et al., 2007; Edward and Dubey, 2013).

New research has show that repeat ovine transmission of *T. gondii* in subsequent pregnancies can occur, unlike previous studies suggest that sheep have aborted due to parasite develop protection against future abortion, although it is believed that has a lower epidemiological importance occurrence, in these animals is possible that reactivation of latent toxoplasmosis can occur and influence in the incidence of infection in sheep (Morley et al. 2005; Innes et al., 2009).

DIAGNOSIS

The suspicion of toxoplasmosis should be raised when abortions are detected in the sheep flock, the placenta should be macroscopically examined, the presence of pinpoint white necrotic foci in the placental caruncles support the preliminary diagnosis, the intercotyledonary region is usually normal or slightly edematous (Dubey, 2010; Gabardo et al., 2013). On post mortem, multiple granulomas may be found in the lungs and the liver, spleen and kidneys may contain areas of necrosis, the central nervous system may contain hemorrhages, edema, ventricular dilatation and areas of inflammation (Mearns, 2007). Veterinarians can perform a rapid diagnosis of toxoplasmosis following the examination of impression smears from the lesions using optical microscope examined for tissue cysts (Dubey et al., 2006; Giadinis et al., 2011). Laboratory confirmation may be established based on mother and fetus serum antibody detection, placental and fetal brain histopathology, immunohistochemistry and PCR (Buxton, 2007).

PREVENTION AND CONTROL

In sheep farm, the main control measure is preventing environmental contamination by oocysts, this requires blocking acess of cats in places where feed is stored, pastures and sources of water (Andrade et al., 2013, Sechi et al., 2013) and controlling stray cat populations on farms (Pavilovic and Ivanovic, 2005). In food sheep productions areas, cats should not be acquired for the purpose of hunting rodents, thus appropriate rodent control is essencial (Jones and Dubey, 2012) and special attention to the using clean or treated water sourcers for the animals (Jones and Dubey, 2012).

T. gondii cannot be macroscopically detected during current meat inspection of livestock while detection methods with high sensitive, practical and inexpensive are not created, prevention remains the best alternative in reducing toxoplasmosis in animals and consequently in man (Bayarry et al., 2012).

Although there a vaccine against toxoplasmosis abortion, however it has not been demonstrated to prevent formation of tecidual cysts, in addition no available drug treatments could completely eliminate *T. gondii* in infected animals, this mean that animals will persistently infected with the parasite (Buxton et al., 1991; Innes et al., 2010), and their efficacy and cost effectiveness for use in infected animals needs to be assessed, this reinforce that prevention is currently the best method to manage the disease in sheep industry.

Treatment protocols for sheep toxoplasmosis are only effective in the acute phase against ovine toxoplasmic abortions, sulfadimidine is commonly used together pyrimethamine (Buxton et al., 1993) or a combination of sulfadimidine and trimethoprim (Buxton and Roger, 2007).

Conclusion

Farmers and veterinarians are the two most important professionals responsible for preventing and controlling of toxoplasmosis and others zoonosis transmitted by consuming food of animal origin (Pritchard, 2011). Thus, should be concerned about the importance of toxoplasmosis; disease that can decisively affect the viability of sheep production and affect public health.

References

Andrade, M. M. C.; Carneiro, M.; Medeiros, A. D.; Andrade Neto, V.; Vitor, R. W. A. 2013. Seroprevalence and risk factors associated with ovine toxoplasmosis in Northeast Brazil. *Parasite*, Vol.20, Nº20, 2013, pp.1-5,1776-1042.

Al-Mabruk, A. A.; Alkhunfas, S. R.; El-Buni, A. A, Annajar, B. B.; Elsaid, M. M. A. 2013. Seroprevalence of *Toxoplasma gondii* antibodies in sheep from Libya. *International Journal of Advanced Research*, Vol.1, N° 9, 2013, pp.148-154, 2320-5407.

Alvarado-Esquivel, C.; Estrada-Malacón, M. A.; Reyes-Hernández, S. O.; Pérez-Ramírez, J. A.; Trujillo-López, J. I.; Villena, I.; Dubey, J. P. 2013. Seroprevalence of *Toxoplasma gondii* in domestic sheep in Oaxaca State, Mexico. *Journal of Parasitology*, Vol. 99, N°1, 2013, pp.151-152, 1937-2345.

Bayarri, S.; Gracia, M. J.; Lázaro, R.; Pérez-Arquillué, C.; Herrera, A. 2012. *Toxoplasma gondii* in Meat and Food Safety Implications - A Review, Zoonosis. Dr. Jacob Lorenzo-Morales (Ed.), ISBN: 978-953-51-0479-7, InTech, Available from: http://www.intechopen.com/ books/zoonosis/ toxoplasma-gondii-in-meat.

Bonfioli, A. A.; Orefice, F. 2005.Toxoplasmosis. Seminars in Ophthalmology, Vol.20, N° 3, 2005, pp.129–141, 0882-0538.

Bresciani, K. D. S.; Galvão, A. L. B.; Vasconcellos, A. L.; Santos, R. R.; Silveira-Neto, L.; Inácio, S. V.; Soares, J. A.; Gomes, J. F.; Santos, T. R. Toxoplasmosis in public health. In: Goodson, B. M; Don Winslow, D. Toxoplasma gondii: Prevalence in Humans and Animals, Genetic Structure and Role in Disease Distribution. New York: Nova Publishers, 2013; pp. 109-122.

Buxton, D.; Thomson, K.; Maley, S.; Wright, S.; Bos ,H. J. 1991. Vaccination of sheep with a live incomplete strain (S48) of *Toxoplasma gondii* and their immunity to challenge when pregnant. *Veterinary Record*, Vol.129, N° 5, 1991, pp.89–93, 0042-4900.

Buxton, D.; Thomson, K. M.; Maley, S. 1993. Treatment of ovine toxoplasmosis with a combination of sulphamezathine and pyrimethamine. *Veterinary Record*, Vol. 132, 1993, pp.409-411, 0042-4900.

Buxton, D.; Rodger, S. M: 2007. Toxoplasmosis and neosporosis. In: Diseases of Sheep, 4th ed., Blackwell Publishing, London, 2007; pp.112-119.

Buxton, D., Maley, S. W., Wright, S. E., Rodger, S., Bartley, P., Innes, E. A., 2007. *Toxoplasma gondii* and ovine toxoplasmosis: new aspects of an old story. *Veterinary Parasitology*, Vol. 149, 2007, pp.25–28, 0304-4017.

Camossi, L. G.; Greca Júnior, H.; Corrêa, A. F. L.; Richini-Pereira, V. B.; Silva, A. V.; Silva, R. C. 2011. Detection of *Toxoplasma gondii* DNA in the Milk of naturally infected ewes. *Veterinary Parasitology*, Vol. 177, N°3, 2011, pp.256-261, 0304-4017.

Cenci Goga, B. T.; Rossitto, P. V.; Sechi, P.; Mc Crindle, C. M. E.; Cullor, J. S. 2011. *Toxoplasma* in animals, food and humans: an old parasite of new concern. *Foodborne Pathogens and Diseases*, Vol. 8, Nº 7, 2011, pp.751-762, 1535-3141.

Cenci Goga, B. T.; Ciampelli, A.; Sechi, P.; Veronesi, F.; Moretta, I.; Cambiotti, V.; Thompson, P. N. 2013. Seroprevalence and risk factors for *Toxoplasma gondii* in sheep in Grosseto district, Tuscany, Italy. BMC *Veterinary Research*, Vol.9, Nº.25, 2013, pp.9, 1746-6148.

Dempster, R. P.; Wilkins, M.; Green, R. S.; de Lisle, G. W. 2011. Serological survey of *Toxoplasma gondii* and *Campylobacter fetus* in sheep from New Zealand. *New Zealand Veterinary Journal*, Vol. 59, Nº.4, 2011, pp.155-159, 0048-0169.

Dubey, J. P.; Hill, D. E.; Jones, J. L.; Hightower, A. W.; Kirkland, E.; Roberts, J. M.; Marcet, P. L.; Lehmann, T.; Vianna, M. C.; Miska, K.; Sreekumar, C.; Kwok, O. C.; Shen, S. K.; Gamble H. R. 2005. Prevalence of viable *Toxoplasma gondii* in beef, chicken, and pork from retail meat stores in the United States: risk assessment to consumers. *The Journal of Parasitology*, Vol.91,Nº.5, 2005, pp.1082–1093, 0022-3395.

Dubey, J. P.; Lindsay, D. S. 2006. Neosporosis, toxoplasmosis and sarcocystosis in ruminants. *Vet. Clin. North America Food Animal Practice,* Vol. 22, Nº. 3, 2006; pp. 645-671, 0749-0720.

Dubey, J. P.; Jones, J. L. 2008. *Toxoplasma gondii* infection in humans and animalsin the United States. *International Journal for Parasitology*, Vol.38, Nº 11, 2008, pp.1257–1278, 0020-7519.

Dubey, J. P. 2009. Toxoplasmosis in sheep – The last 20 years. *Veterinary Parasitology*, Vol. 163, Nº 1-2, 2009, pp.1-14, 0304-4017.

Dubey, J. P. 2010. Toxoplasmosis of Animals and Humans. Second Edition. CRC Press Taylor and Francis Group. 978-1-4200-9236-3. 313p.

Edwards, J. F.; Dubey, J. P. 2013. *Toxoplasma gondii* abortion storm in sheep on a Texas farm and isolation of mouse virulent atypical genotype *T. gondii* from an aborted lamb from a chronically infected ewe. *Veterinary Parasitology,* Vol.192, , Nº 1-2, 2013, pp. 129– 136, 0304-4017.

EFSA. 2013. Technical specifications on harmonised epidemiological indicators for biological hazards to be covered by meat inspection of domestic sheep and goats. *European Food Safety Authority (EFSA) Journal,* Vol. 11, Nº. 6, 2013, 66p.

Fusco, G.; Rinaldi, L.; Guarino, A.; Proroga, Y.; Pesce, A.; Giuseppina de, M.; Cringoli, G. 2007. *Toxoplasma gondii* in sheep from the Campania region (Italy). *Veterinary Parasitology*, Vol.149, Nº.3-4, 2007, pp.271–274, 0304-4017.

Gabardo, M. P.; Oliveira, J. S. V.; Ecco, R.; Guedes, R. M. C. 2013.

Outbreak of ovine abortion by Toxoplasmosis in Southeastern. 2013. *Brazilian Journal Veterinary Pathology*, Vol.6, N°.1, 2013, pp.37-41, 1983-0246.

Gangneux, F. R.; Dardé, M. L. 2012. Epidemiology of and diagnostic strategies for Toxoplasmosis. *Clinical Microbiology Reviews*, Vol.25, N°.2, 2012, pp.64, 0893-8512.

García-Bocanegra, I.; Cabezón, O.; Hernández, E.; Martínez-Cruz, M. S.; Martínez-Moreno, Á.; Martínez-Moreno, J. Toxoplasma gondii in ruminant species (cattle, sheep, and goats) from southern Spain. *The Journal of Parasitology,* Vol.99, N°.3, pp.438-440, 1937-2345.

Gebremedhin, E. Z.; Agonafir, A.; Tessema, T. S.; Tilahun, G.; Medhin, G.; Vitale, M.; Di Marco, V.; Cox, E.; Vercruysse, J.; Dorny, P. 2013. Seroepidemiological study of ovine toxoplasmosis in East and West Shewa Zones of Oromia Regional State, Central Ethiopia. *BMC Veterinary Research,* Vol.9:117, 2013, pp.1-8, 1746-6148.

Giadinis, N. D.; Terpsidis, K.; Diakou, A.; Siarkou, V.; Loukopoulos, P.; Osman, R.; Karatzias, H.; Papazahariadou, M. 2011. Massive *toxoplasma* abortions in a dairy sheep flock and therapeutic approach with different doses of sulfadimidine. *Turkish Journal of Veterinary and Animal Science,* Vol. 35, N°.3, 2011, pp. 207-211, 1300-0128.

Halová, D.; Mulcahy, G.; Rafter, P.; Turčeková, L.; Grant, T.; de Waal, T. 2013. *Toxoplasma gondii* in Ireland: seroprevalence and novel molecular detection method in sheep, pigs, deer and chickens. *Zoonoses Public Health,* Vol.60, N°.2, 2013, pp.168-173, 1863-1959.

Hecker, Y. P.; Moore, D. P.; Manazza, J. A.; Unzaga, J. M.; Späth, E. J.; Pardini, L. L.; Venturini, M. C.; Roberi, J. L.; Campero, C. M. 2013. First report of seroprevalence of *Toxoplasma gondii* and *Neospora caninum* in dairy sheep from Humid Pampa, Argentina. *Tropical Animal Health and Production,* Vol. 45, N°.7, 2013, pp.1645-1647, 0049-4747.

Heidari, H.; Gharekhani, J.; Tavoosidana, G. 2013. Role of toxoplasmosis in abortion of ewes in western Iran: a serological study. *Science Parasitology,* Vol 14, N°.2, 2013, pp. 99-103, 1582-1366.

Innes. E. A.; Vermeulen, A. N. 2006.Vaccination as a control strategy against the coccidial parasites *Eimeria*, *Toxoplasma* and *Neospora*. *Parasitology,* Vol.133, N°.S2, 2006, pp.145–168, 0031-1820.

Innes, E. A.; Bartley, P. M.; Buxton, D.; Katzer, F. 2009. Ovine Toxoplasmosis. *Parasitology*, Vol.136, N°.14, 2009, pp.1887-1894, 0031-1820.

Innes, E. A. 2010.Vaccination against *Toxoplasma gondii*: an increasing priority for collaborative research? *Expert Review Vaccines*, Vol.9, Nº. 10, 2010, pp.1117–1119, 1476-0584.

Jones, J. L.; Dubey, J. P. 2012. Foodborne toxoplasmosis: Food Safety. *Clinical Infectious Diseases Advance Access,* Vol.55, Nº.6, 2012, pp.845-851, 1058-4838.

Kortbeek, L. M.; Hofhuis, A.; Nijhuis, C. D.; Havelaar, A. H. 2009. Congenital toxoplasmosis and DALYs in the Netherlands. *Memórias do Instituto Oswaldo Cruz,* Vol. 104, Nº.2, 2009, pp.370-373, 0074-0276.

Lopes, A. P.; Dubey, J. P.; Neto, F.; Rodrigues, A.; Martins, T.; Rodrigues, M.; Cardoso L. 2013. Seroprevalence of *Toxoplasma gondii* infection in cattle, sheep, goats and pigs from the North of Portugal for human consumption. *Veterinary Parasitology*, Vol. 193, Nº. 1-3, 2013, pp.266-269, 0074-0276. 0304-4017.

McColgan, C.; Buxton, D.; Blewett, D. 1988. Titration of *Toxoplasma gondii* oocysts in non-pregnant sheep and the effects of subsequent challenge during pregnancy. *The Veterinary Record*, Vol.123, Nº.18, 1988, pp.467-470, 0042-4900.

Mearns, R. 2007. Abortion in sheep: Investigation and principal causes. Clinical Practice: Farm Animal Practice. *In Practice*, Vol. 29, Nº.1, 2007, pp.40-46, 0263/841 X.

Morley, E.; Williams, R.; Hughes, J.; Terry, R.; Duncanson, P. 2005. Significant familial differences in the frequency of abortion and *Toxoplasma gondii* infection within a flock of Charollais sheep. *Parasitology,* Vol. 131, Nº.2, 2005, pp.181-185, 0031-1820.

Pavlovic, I.; Ivanovic, S. 2005. Toxoplasmosis of goats and its role and importance in pathology of goat production. *Biotechonology in Animal Husbandry*, Vol. 21, Nº.5-6, 2005, pp.123-126, 1450-9156.

Pritchard, G. Prevention and control of zoonoses on farms open to the public. 2011. Clinical Practice. *Farm Animal Practice*, Vol. 33, 2011, pp.242-251, 2042-7689.

Scallan, E.; Hoekstra, R. M.; Angulo, F. J.; Tauxe, R. V.; Widdowson, M. A.; Roy, S. L.; Jones, J. L.; Griffin, P. M. 2011. Foodborne Illness adquired in the United States -Major Pathogens. *Emerging Infections Diseases,* Vol.17, Nº. 1, 2011, pp.7-15, 1880-6040.

Sechi, P.; Ciampelli, A.; Cambiotti, V.; Veronezi, F.; Cenci-Goga, B. T. 2013. Seroepidemiological study of toxoplasmosis in sheep in rural areas of the Grosseto district, Tuscany, Italy. 2013. *Italian Journal of Animal Science,* Vol.12, Nº. 39, 2013, pp.236-239, 1594-4077.

Veterinary Investigation Diagnosis Analysis (VIDA). Yearly Trends 2002-2009 for sheep. [http://vla.defra.gov.uk/reports/docs/rep_vida_sheep02_09.pdf]

Yang, N.; Li, H.; He, J.; Mu, M.; Yang, S. 2013. Seroprevalence of Toxoplasma gondii infection in domestic sheep in Liaoning Province, northeastern China. *The Journal of Parasitology*, Vol.99, Nº. 1, 2013, pp.174-175, 1937-2345.

In: Recent Advances in Toxoplasmosis Research ISBN: 978-1-63117-914-3
Editor: Connor M. Lee

Chapter 7

NEONATAL TOXOPLASMOSIS IN DOGS AND KITTENS

Katia Denise Saraiva Bresciani[1,2,*], André Luiz Baptista Galvão[2], Amanda Leal de Vasconcelllos[2], Lucas Vinicius Shigaki de Matos[2], Julia Cestari Pierucci[2], Marion Burkhardt de Koivisto[1], Claudio Alessandro Masamtsu Sakamoto[2], José Antonio Soares[3], Thais Rabelo dos Santos[4] and Alvimar José da Costa[2]

[1]UNESP, Universidade Estadual Paulista Júlio de Mesquita Filho, Faculdade de Medicina Veterinária de Araçatuba, Araçatuba, São Paulo, Brazil

[2]UNESP, Universidade Estadual Paulista Júlio de Mesquita Filho, Faculdade de Ciências Agrárias e Veterinárias, Jaboticabal, São Paulo, Brazil

[3]Faculdades Integradas de Itapetininga, Fundação Karnig Bazarian, Itapetininga, São Paulo, Brazil

[4]UNIR, Fundação Universidade Federal de Rondônia, Departamento de Medicina Veterinária, Campus de Rolim de Moura, Rolim de Moura, Rondônia, Brazil

[*] E-mail: bresciani@fmva.unesp.br.

Abstract

The protozoan parasite *Toxoplasma gondii* commonly infects cats, dogs and humans. Toxoplasmosis is an important issue concerning public health, particularly involving the risk of disease transmission during pregnancy. The infection can be acquired by ingestion of tissue cysts in infected meat, ingestion of food or water contaminated with oocysts and congenitally, by tachyzoites crossing the placenta from the infected mother to the fetus. Congenital *T. gondii* infection has been reported in many species of animals. The organism strain, dose, and the stage of fetal development or age of the host at the time of infection likely influence the presence or severity of clinical toxoplasmosis in the neonate. The infecting stage of the organism (tachyzoite, oocyst, cyst) may also be important. Uterine changes were observed in bitches with toxoplasmosis (endometritis). Cats with disseminated organism replication which in clinical toxoplasmosis usually have multiple organ involvement that commonly includes the eyes. Ocular toxoplasmosis can occur without other evidence of clinical illness in kittens infected in uterus or in the neonatal period, and *T. gondii* strains may have varying degrees of ocular pathogenicity in cats. The aim of this chapter will be to elucidate some clinical neonatal aspects in view of congenital toxoplasmosis in cat and dog.

Introduction

Toxoplasmosis in children leads to severe damage to fetuses producing diffuse necrotizing encephalitis despite some periventricular lesions of hydrocephalus have been reported (Wolf and Cowen, 1968). This is an important issue which concerns public health, particularly involving the risk of disease transmission during pregnancy when undergo miscarriage, premature birth, neonatal death and even the classical Sabin's Triad, characterized by retinochoroiditis, cerebral calcifications, hydrocephaly or microcephaly (Jones et al., 2001; Soares et al., 2011; Navarro et al., 2013; Bresciani et al., 2013a; Bresciani et al., 2013b; Bresciani et al., 2014; Doudou et al., 2014).

Severe cases of congenital toxoplasmosis occurs with greater frequency when the mother is infected during the first two trimesters of pregnancy, but when the disease is acquired later, symptoms tend to be subclinical or even absent in the fetus (Bayat et al., 2013).

In small animals, the infection has been reported in several countries, leading to varied clinical uncommon manifestations, but severe and fatal, which is a challenge in the clinical diagnosis of small animals, especially with the nervous system involvement (Lavely, 2013, Galvão et al., 2014).

Cats may disseminate in the environment *Toxoplasma gondii* faecal oocysts (Frenkel et al., 1970) acting as intermediate or definitive hosts (Dubey et al., 1995). The toxoplasmic infection can be also acquired by ingestion of tissue cysts in infected meat (Dubey and Beattle, 1988), and congenitally, by tachyzoites crossing the placenta from the infected mother to the fetus (Elsheikha, 2008). A higher tendency of *T. gondii* occurance was noted for young cats, which had access to the external environment, cohabited with mice, and fed with homemade food and raw milk. It was observed that the parasite is probably linked to postnatal infection in association with the type of diet and presence of rats (Coelho et al., 2011).

Although there is the possibility of perpetuation of *T. gondii* cycle in the absence of cats, it seems that this species is of essential importance in the transmission of toxoplasmosis in different locations worldwide (Bresciani et al., 2013c). Additionally, dogs play a important role in the transmission of oocysts to humans (Lindsay et al., 1997) that can be mechanically shed or transported by dogs, thereby contaminating the environment (Jittapalapong et al., 2007, Bresciani et al., 2013d).

Considering the close proximity between men (mainly children and old people) and pets and the zoonotic potential of the toxoplasmosis, the study of this disease in pets has become interesting. Thus, the purpose of this review is to discuss the clinical aspects of neonatal toxoplasmosis in dogs and cats.

Congenital Transmission of *Toxoplasma gondii* in Dogs

In reports of *Toxoplasma* encephalitis in neonatal or young dogs the infection has not been associated with acquired hydrocephalus. This protozoan can cause severe damage to infected fetuses during pregnancy (Hartley et al., 1958; Higgins et al., 1977).

It was demonstrated that *T. gondii* can be congenitally transmitted in dogs when bitches are infected during pregnancy (Bresciani et al., 1999). Fever, nasal discharge, tearing, prostration, lymphadenopathy, premature birth, spontaneous abortion, fetal death, miscarriage and stillbirth were found in pregnant dogs infected by this parasite (Bresciani et al., 1999; Bresciani et al., 2001). It is worth highlighting that after the primary experimental infection whith *T. gondii* oocysts and tachyzoites in female dogs, this parasite was detected in samples of saliva, milk and urine by bioassay in mice (Bresciani et al., 2001). This infection is a proven cause of reproductive failures in canines (Smielewska et al., 2003).

Also, in a study of toxoplasmic reinfection during pregnancy, the fetuses were born apparently healthy but seropositive. The *T.gondii* was detected by imunohistochemistry in the encephalon of a neonate and in the spinal cord of a stillborn, thus confirming that *T. gondii* infected canine fetuses, leading to uterine changes miscarriages, even in bitches that presented primo infection (Bresciani et al., 2009).

Presence of *T. gondii* in semen, testicles and epididymis in male dogs with experimental toxoplasmosis was described. Seven days after inoculation of PCR-positive for the parasite seminal samples, female dogs with negative titration showed serologic conversion. Fetal resorption was also evidenced during pregnancy and toxoplasmic cysts were found in the encephalon of pupies, confirming the sexual transmission of this infection (Arantes et al., 2009).

The concomitant infections of *Canine distemper virus* (CDV), *Canine adenovirus A* types 1 (CAdV-1) and 2 (CAdV-2), Canine parvovirus type 2 (CPV-2), and *Toxoplasma gondii* were described in a 43-day-old mixed-breed puppy. Clinically, there were convulsions and blindness with spontaneous death; 14 siblings of this puppy, born to a 10-month old dam, which was seropositive (titer: 1,024) for *T. gondii*, also died. The PCR assays demonstrated that the apicomplexan protozoa observed within several organs contained DNA specific for *T. gondii*; genotyping revealed *T. gondii* type III. Further, seroreactivity to *T. gondii* of the dam in association with the systemic disease observed in the puppy described herein is suggestive of congenital toxoplasmosis (Headley et al., 2013).

Congenital Transmission of *Toxoplasma gondii* in Cats

Ocular toxoplasmosis can occur without other evidence of clinical illness in kittens infected in uterus or in the neonatal period, and that *T. gondii* strains may have varying degrees of ocular pathogenicity in cats (Powell and Lappin, 2001). Kittens infected via placenta or lactogenic ways may show inflammatory processes that affect the liver, lungs and central nervous system, which reflects clinically as uveitis, lethargy, depression, ascites, encephalitis, hypothermia and sudden death (Dubey and Lappin, 2006).

Transmission during lactation has been considered the most common transmission route in cats instead of the placenta via. The quantity of serum antibody acquired by kittens through colostrum decreases after the first 15 days of age and disappears around 10 weeks of age (Dubey et al., 1995). Animals that were up to 15-day-old and less than 60-day-old are carriers of specific antibodies to *T. gondii*, suggesting that the infection occurred either intra-uterine or antibodies were acquired through colostrum (Svoboda and Svobodová, 1987, Bresciani et al., 2007, Cardia et al., 2013).

Abortion and neonatal mortality were described in pregnant queens orally inoculated with tissue cysts from different strains of undefined *T. gondii* genotype (Dubey and Hoover, 1977; Sato et al., 1993; Dubey and Carpenter, 1993; Dubey et al., 1995; Dubey, 1996; Powel et al., 2001). The infection caused by tachyzoites of *T. gondii* from maternal milk has been reported in the literature (Powell et al., 2001).

If the queen has systemic toxoplasmosis, it may abort due to systemic illness rather than direct fetal infection (Pretzer, 2008). Transplacental transmission and fetal infection with *T gondii* have been shown in experimentally infected cats and has been associated with fetal death. The pathogenicity of two major brazilian lineages was investigated after oral inoculation of queens in the middle third of their pregnancies with *T. gondii* cysts. The infection with type BrI isolate causes toxoplasmosis manifestations and abortion from one litter. Toxoplasmosis manifestations besides premature stillbirth of one litter were observed in queens with type BrIII isolate (Sakamoto et al., 2009).

Conclusion

By this way, in this chapter some clinical neonatal aspects due to congenital toxoplasmosis in pets were exposed.

References

Arantes , T. P.; Lopes , W. D,; Ferreira , R. M.; Pieroni , J. S.; Pinto, V. M.; Sakamoto, C. A.; Costa, A. J. *Toxoplasma gondii* : evidências para a transmissão de sêmen em cães . *Experimental Parasitology*, 2009, vol. 123, pp. 190 - 194.

Bayat, P. D.; Eslamirad, Z.; Shojaee, S. Toxoplasmosis: experimental vaginal infections in NMRI mice and its effect on uterin, placenta and fetus tissues. *Irian Red Crescent Medical Journal*, 2013, vol. 15, pp. 595-599.

Bresciani, K. D. S.; Costa, A. J.; Toniollo, G. H.; Sabatini, G. A.; Moraes, F. R.; Paulilo, A. C.; Ferraudo, A. S. Experimental toxoplasmosis in pregnant bitches. *Veterinary Parasitology*, 1999, vol. 86, pp. 143-145.

Bresciani, K. D. S.; Toniollo, G. H.; Costa, A. J.; Sabatini, G. A.; Moraes, F. R. Clinical, parasitological and obstetric observations in pregnant bitches with experimental toxoplasmosis, *Ciência Rural*, 2001, vol. 31, pp. 1039-1043.

Bresciani, K. D. S.; Costa, A. J.; Toniollo, G. H.; Luvizotto, M. C. R.; Kanamura, T.; Moraes, F. R.; Perri, S. H. V.; Gennari, S. M. Transplacental transmission of *Toxoplasma gondii* in reinfected pregnant female canines. *Parasitology Research*, 2009, vol. 104, pp. 1213-1217.

Bresciani K. D. S.; Galvão, A. B. G.; Vasconcellos, A. L.; Soares, J. A.; Matos, L. V. S.; Pierucci, J. C.; Silveira-Neto, L.; Rodrigues, T. O.; Navarro, I. T.; Costa, A. J. Relevant aspects of human toxoplasmosis. *Research Journal of Infectious Diseases*, 2013a, vol. 2, n. 4, pp. 114-118.

Bresciani, K. D. S.; Galvão, A. L. B.; Vasconcellos, A. L.; Santos, R. R.; Silveira-Neto, L.; Inácio, S. V.; Soares, J. A.; Gomes, J. F.; Santos, T. R. Toxoplasmosis in public health. In: Goodson, BM; Don Winslow, D. *Toxoplasma gondii*: Prevalence in Humans and Animals, Genetic Structure and Role in Disease Distribution. New York: Nova Publishers, 2013c; pp. 109-122.

Bresciani, K. D. S.; Camossi, L. G., Cardia, D. F. F.; Soares,J. Á.; Teixeira,W. F. P.; Santos,T. R.; Neto, L. S.; Matos, L. V. S.; Gomes, J. F.; Costa, A. J. Need for a continuing education program for canine toxoplasmosis control. *Main Canine Protozoan Zoonosis*, 2014.

Bresciani, K. D. S.; Galvão, A. L. B.; Vasconcellos, A. L.; Gomes, J. F.; Santos, T. R.; Santos, R. R.; Viol, M. A.; Aquino, M. C. C.; Navarro, I. T. Epidemiology and control of toxoplasmosis in cats. In: Goodson, BM; Don Winslow, D. *Toxoplasma gondii:* Prevalence in Humans and Animals, Genetic Structure and Role in Disease Distribution. New York: Nova Publishers, 2013c; pp. 95-108.

Bresciani, K. D. S.; Galvão, A. L. B.; Vasconcellos, A. L.; Navarro, I. T.; Gomes, J. F.; Santos, R. R.; Santos, T. R.; Costa, A. J. Epidemiology and control of toxoplasmosis in dogs. In: Goodson, B. M; Don Winslow, D.

Toxoplasma gondii: Prevalence in Humans and Animals, Genetic Structure and Role in Disease Distribution. New York: Nova Publishers, 2013d; pp. 43-60.

Cardia, D. F. F; Camossi, L. G; Neto, L. S.; Langoni,H.; Bresciani, K. D. S. Prevalence of *Toxoplasma gondii* and *Leishmania* spp. Infection in cats from Brazil. *Veterinary Parasitology*, 2013, vol. 197, pp. 634– 637.

Coelho, W. M. D.; Amarante, A. F. T.; Apolinário, J. C.; Coelho, N. M. D.; Lima, V. M. F.; Perri, S. H. V.; Bresciani, K. D. S., Seroepidemiology of *Toxoplasma gondii, Neospora caninum* and *Leishmania spp*. infections and risk factors for cats from Brazil. *Parasitology Research,* 2011, vol. 109, n. 4, pp. 1009–1013.

Doudou, Y.; Renaud,P.; Coralie, L. O.; Jacqueline, F.; Hypolite, S.; Hypolite, M.; Patrick, M.; Andreia, I. L. R.; Marc,V. S.; Marleen, B.; Pierre, V. G. J.; Pascal, L. Toxoplasmosis among pregnant women: High seroprevalence and risk factors in Kinshasa, Democratic Republic of Congo. *Asian Pacific Journal of Tropical Biomedicine*, 2014, vol. 4, n.1, pp. 69-74.

Dubey, J. P.; Hoover, E. A. Attempted transmission of *Toxoplasma gondii* infection form pregnant cats to their kittens. *Journal American Veterinary Medical Association,* 1977, vol. 170, pp. 538-540.

Dubey, J. P.; Beattle, C. P. Toxoplasmosis of animals and man, *CRC, Boca Raton*, 1988.

Dubey, J. P.; Carpenter, J. L. Unidentified Toxoplasma like tissue cysts in the brains of three cats. *Veterinary Parasitology, Amsterdam*, 1993, vol. 45, pp. 319-321.

Dubey, J. P.; Lappin, M. R.; Thulliez, M. Diagnosis of induced toxoplasmosis in neonatal cats. *Journal of American Veterinary Medical Association*, 1995, vol. 207, pp. 179-185.

Dubey, J. P. Strategies to reduce transmission of *Toxoplasma gondii* to animals and humans. *Veterinary Parasitology*, 1996, vol. 64, pp. 65-70.

Dubey, J. P.; Lappin, M. R. Toxoplasmosis and Neosporosis. In Infectious Diseases of the Dog and Cat; C. E. Greene ,W. B. Saunders, Philadelphia, 2006, n. 2, pp. 754-775.

Elsheikha, H. M. Congenital toxoplasmosis: priorities for further health promotion action. *Public Health*, 2008, vol. 122, pp. 335-353.

Frenkel, J. K, Dubey, J. P., Miller, N. L. *Toxoplasmosis gondii* in cats: fecal stages indentified as coccidian oocysts. *Science,* 1970, vol. 167, pp. 893-896.

Galvão, A. L. B.; Vaconcellos, A. L.; Navarro, I. T.; Bresciani, K. D. S. Clinical aspects of toxoplasmosis in small animal. *Semina: Ciências Agrárias, Londrina*, 2014, vol. 35, n. 1, pp. 393-410. DOI: 10.5433/1679-0359.2014v35n1p393

Hartley, W. J.; Lindsay, A. B.; Mackinnon, M. M. Toxoplasma meningo-encephalomyelitis and myositis in a dog. *New Zealand Veterinary Journal*, 1958, vol. 6, pp. 124-127.

Headley, S. A.; Alfieri, A. F.; Fritzen, J. T. T.; Garcia,J. L.; Weissenböck,H.; Silva, A. P.; Bodnar,L.; Okano, W.; Alfieri, A. A. Concomitant canine distemper, infectious canine hepatitis, canine parvoviral enteritis, canine infectious tracheobronchitis, and toxoplasmosis in a puppy. *Journal of Veterinary Diagnostic Investigation,* 2013, DOI: 10.1177/1040638712471344.

Higgins, R. J.; Vandervelde, M.; Braund, B. Internal Hydrocephalus and associated periventricular encephalitis in young dog, *Veterinary Pathology*, 1977, vol. 14, pp. 236-246.

Jittapalapong, S.; Burin, N.; Nongnuch, P.; Chimnoi, W.; Kabeya, H.; Maruyama, S. Seroprevalence of *Toxoplasma gondii* antibodies in stray cats and dogs in the Bangkok metropolitan area, Thailand, *Veterinary Parasitology*, 2007, vol. 145, pp. 138-141.

Jones, J. L., Kruszon-Moran, D.; Wilson, M.; McQuillan, G.; Navin, T.; McAuley, J. B: *Toxoplasma gondii* infection in the United States: Seroprevalence and Risk Factors. *American Journal of Epidemiology,* 2001, vol. 154, pp. 357-365.

Lavely, J. A. Pediatric Seizure Disorders in Dogs and Cats. Veterinary Clinics of North America: Small Animal Practice, 2013 (in press).

Lindsay, D. S.; Dubey, J. P.; Butler, J. M.; Blagburn, B. L. Mechanical transmission of *Toxoplasma gondii* oocysts by dogs. *Veterinary Parasitology*, 1997, vol. 73, pp. 27-33.

Navarro, I. T.; Breganó, R. M.; Mori, F. M. R. L.; Rodrigues, T. O.; Santos, T. R.; Bresciani, K. D. S. *Control program of congenital toxoplasmosis. Toxoplasma gondii*: prevalence in humans and animals, genetic structure and role in disease distribution. New York: Nova Publishers, 2013.

Powell, C. C.; Brewer, M.; Lappin, M. R. Detection of *Toxoplasma gondii* in the milk of experimentally infected lactating cats. *Veterinary Parasitology*, 2001, vol. 102, pp. 29-33.

Powell, C. C.; Lapppin, M. R. Clinical ocular toxoplasmosis in neonatal kittens. *Veterinary Ophthalmology*, 2001, vol. 4, n. 2, pp. 87-92.

Pretzer, S. D. Bacterial and protozoal causes of pregnancy loss in the bitch and queen. *Theriogenology,* 2008, vol. 70, pp. 320–326.

Sakamoto, C. A. M.; Costa, A. J.; Gennari, S. M.; Pena, H. F. J.; Toniollo, G. H.; Lopes, W. D. Z.; Bichuette, M. A.; Betini, C. M.; Amarante, A. F. T.; Bresciani, K. D. S. Experimental infection of pregnant queens with two major Brazilian clonal lineages of *Toxoplasma gondii. Parasitology Research*, 2009, vol. 105, n. 5, pp. 1311-1316.

Sato, K.; Iwamoto, I.; Yoshike, K. Experimental toxoplasmosis in pregnant cats. *Journal Veterinary Medicine Science*, 1993, vol. 55, pp. 1005-1009.

Smielewska, L. E.; Rypula, K.; Dzimira, S. Studies on congenital toxoplasmosis in canines. *Medycyna Wet*, 2003, vol. 59, pp. 141-145.

Soares, J. A. S.; Násser, L. S.; Carvalho, S. F. G.; Caldeira, A. P. Achados oculares em crianças com toxoplasmose congênita. *Arquivos Brasileiros de Oftalmologia,* 2011, vol. 74, pp. 255-257.

Svoboda, M.; Svobodová, V. Effects of breed, sex, age, management and nutrition on the incidence of *Toxoplasma gondii* antibodies in dogs and cats. *Acta Veterinaria Brno*, 1987, vol. 56, pp. 315-330.

Wolf, A.; Cowen, D. Perinatal infections of the central nervous system. Pathologic of the nervous system, McGraw-Hill, New York, 1968, vol. 3, pp. 2565-2611.

In: Recent Advances in Toxoplasmosis Research ISBN: 978-1-63117-914-3
Editor: Connor M. Lee

Chapter 8

DEVELOPMENT OF VECTOR VACCINES AGAINST *TOXOPLASMA GONDII* INFECTION

***Longzheng Yu*[1, 2], *Gabriel Oluga Aboge*[1, 3], *Shoufa Zhang*[2] and *Xuenan Xuan*[1, *]**

[1]National Research Center for Protozoan Diseases, Obihiro University of Agriculture and Veterinary Medicine, Inada-cho, Obihiro, Hokkaido, Japan
[2]Department of Veterinary Medicine, Agricultural College of Yanbian University, Gongyuan Road, Yanji, Jilin, China
[3]Department of Public Health, Pharmacology and Toxicology, University of Nairobi, Kangemi, Nairobi, Kenya

ABSTRACT

Toxoplasma gondii is an obligate intracellular parasite belonging to the phylum Apicomplexa, infecting all warm-blooded animals, with a worldwide distribution. Effective vaccines may contribute toward preventing and controlling the spread of toxoplasmosis. At present, only one commercial vaccine based on the live-attenuated S48 strain was developed for sheep and goats, while a vaccine for pigs, cats and humans is still lacking. Therefore, the focus of current review is to identify the protective antigens and develop antigen delivery systems. Searching the

* Corresponding Author: Dr. Xuenan Xuan. National Research Center for Protozoan Diseases, Obihiro University of Agriculture and Veterinary Medicine, Inada-cho, Obihiro, Hokkaido 080-8555, Japan. Tel: +81 155 49 5648. Fax: +81 155 49 5643. E-mail: gen@obihiro.ac.jp.

undiscovered vaccine candidates by genomics, transcriptomics, and proteomics is an effective approach.

On the other hand, many effective vaccine carriers have been investigated for their ability to induce a wide range of protective immune responses including humoral and cellular immunity, as well as protective effect.

This article presents the current status of vaccine strategies against toxoplasmosis, with a focus on the most advanced approaches using DNA-, virus- and protozoa-based vector vaccines.

INTRODUCTION

Toxoplasma gondii is an obligate intracellular protozoan parasite that can infect warm-blooded vertebrate and humans (Tenter, 2000). *T. gondii* has a complex life cycle consisting of a sexual cycle in its feline definitive hosts and an asexual cycle in its intermediate host. There are four invasive forms of *T. gondii*: the tachyzoite, bradyzoite, merozoite, and sporozoite. Tachyzoites and bradyzoites are associated with the intermediate host, and merozoites and sporozoites with the definitive host (Ferguson, 2007; Dubey, 2009). Tachyzoites and merozoites are responsible for the expansion of the population within a host, while the bradyzoites and sporozoites are capable of environmental transmission to new hosts (Ferguson, 2007). Hosts can acquire *T. gondii* by ingesting either tissues of infected animals or food or drink contaminated with sporulated oocysts, or by transplacental transmission (Dubey, 2008).

After ingestion, bradyzoites released from tissue cysts or sporozoites from oocysts penetrate intestinal tissues, transform to tachyzoites, and are disseminated throughout the body via blood or lymph (Dubey, 2004). In response to the host's immune system, the tachyzoites multiply asexually and produce cysts, which contain the bradyzoites (Brown, 1994). When the immune system becomes compromised, the bradyzoites can convert to tachyzoites, and tachyzoites are highly virulent and cause a generalized toxoplasmosis (Weiss, 2000).

Infection in domestic animals is a threat to public health from food-borne outbreaks and causes a great economic loss as it may lead to abortion, stillbirth and neonatal loss (Jones, 2012). Treatment of this disease is difficult since the available drugs have severe side effects and reactivation may occur at any time (Montoya, 2004). Therefore, developing an effective vaccine against *T. gondii* infection is desired.

Host Immune Responses in *Toxoplasma Gondii* Infection

Immunity to *T. gondii* is complex, with aspects of innate and adaptive immune response playing important effectors roles (Gazzinelli, 1992). When intermediate hosts ingest tissue cysts or oocysts containing *T. gondii*, free parasites are released in the gut lumen (Courret, 2006). When enterocytes are infected by the parasites, enterocytes may secrete cytotoxic molecules such as nitric oxide (NO) (Buzoni-Gatel, 2006). In addition, enterocytes respond to the infection by secretion of chemokines and cytokines, which attract polymorphonuclear leukocytes (PMNs), macrophages, natural killer (NK) cells, and dendritic cells (DCs) (Buzoni-Gatel, 2006). *T. gondii* can efficiently enter and survive within nucleated cells, such as DCs, and the functional migratory property of DCs can be utilized by pathogens for dissemination through the body (Channon, 2000). When stimulated, these cells from the innate immune system can be directly microbicidal (Buzoni-Gatel, 2006). These cells of the innate immune system are also source of cytokines such as interleukin (IL)-12 and interferon gamma (IFN-γ), and the two cytokines are central to control the replication of *T. gondii* (Courret, 2006).

Cytokines play a crucial role against *T. gondii* infection. IFN-γ, IL-12, IL-18, and TNF-α (tumor necrosis factor-alpha) produced by NK cells, DCs, and monocytes directly limit acute infection and lead to the differentiation of antigen-specific CD4+ T-cells into Th1 effector T-cells that produce more IFN-γ. The IFN-γ produced indoleamine 2,3-dioxygenase (IDO) and inducible nitric oxide synthase (iNOS) in target cells, which are effective in inhibiting and killing *T. gondii* tachyzoites (Scharton-Kersten, 1997). Cytolytic $CD8^{+}$ T-cells recognize specific *T. gondii*-derived peptides by major histocompatibility complex (MHC) I molecule, and can also kill target cells by release of perforin and granzyme (Roberts, 2007). Cytokines may lead to evasion of initial activation of protective immunity or curtail a potentially lethal immune response (Neyer, 1997). For example, in the absence of IL-10, the inflammatory process is lethal. Presence of IL-4 early in infection inhibits protective Th1 responses, but later inhibits *Toxoplasma* replication within central nervous system (CNS).

Thus, the temporal sequence of cytokine production is important (Bourguin, 1993). The relative balance between Th1 and Th2 cytokines appears to be crucial in a protective immune response against infection by *T. gondii* (Yu, 2012).

Antibodies are involved in resistance against *T. gondii,* although cellular immunity plays a major role. B cells are triggered to secrete antibodies to provide protection against *T. gondii* infection (Casadevall, 2006). Frenkel and Taylor examined the effect of depletion of B cells on toxoplasmosis in mice infected with a virulent strain (Frenkel, 1982). They observed mortality associated with antibodies. Administration of antiserum to *T. gondii* reduces mortality in animal model. These results suggest that antibodies production by B cells may be important for controlling the latent persistent infection. More recently, Sayles et al. have demonstrated that antibodies directed against surface antigens may prevent infection of host cells (Sayles, 2000). Kang et al. (2000) reported the role of B cells in resistance to *T. gondii* that mice lacking B cells showed that those animals are susceptible to chronic infection and are not protected after vaccination. Johnson and Sayles reported that treatment of CD4-deficient mice with anti-*T. gondii* sera prolonged their survival during the chronic stage of infection (Johnson, 2002). These results indicate that B cell play an important role, through production of specific antibodies.

The Current Status of Development of Vaccines Against *Toxoplasma gondii Infection*

A successful vaccine would have beneficial impacts in both medical and veterinary fields. For the control of *T. gondii* infection in host, vaccination is generally considered to be the most effective means to control and alleviate *T. gondii* infection. However, at present, only the attenuated S48 strain was developed to a commercial vaccine for use in sheep and goats (Wilkins, 1988). In 1988, it was introduced as Toxovax®, a live vaccine, in New Zealand. This commercial vaccine has the possibility of reverting to pathogenicity. In addition, this commercially available *Toxoplasma* vaccine only provides protection in sheep and goat, while a vaccine for humans and other animals is still lacking (Innes, 2009). In search of a safe and efficacious vaccine against toxoplasmosis, different strategies including the use of live attenuated parasites, gene deletion attenuated parasites, bacterial vector vaccines, viral vector vaccines, protozoan vector vaccines, DNA vaccines, and subunit vaccines etc. have been reported to induce significant humoral and cellular immune response (Jongert, 2009). Overall, some vaccines increased survival following challenge infection, but not sterile immunity. Therefore, the focus of current research is to identify the protective antigens and then present them to the immune system and determine an appropriate antigen delivery system to stimulate appropriate protective immunity.

SEARCHING FOR NOVEL VACCINE CANDIDATES

Due to complex life cycle involving multiple hosts with diversity of protein expression and variety of invasion pathways, *T. gondii* exhibits a very high degree of antigenic polymorphism and variability. Although several candidate antigens have been identified in the past few years, the ones capable of inducing a strong and long-lasting protective immunity are limited. Therefore, selection of target antigens is a crucial step to design effective vaccines (Innes, 2006).

Proteomics is a useful tool for obtaining a more complete understanding of the biology of parasites (Belli, 2005). Protein expression analysis using two-dimensional electrophoresis (2-DE) technologies combined with immunoblot analysis and then coupled with matrix-assisted laser desorption/ionization–time-of-flight mass spectrometry (MALDI-TOF MS) provides a means to identify parasite-specific proteins and antigenic proteins that represent potential vaccine candidates (Klade, 2002). Cohen et al. (2002) characterized a 2-DE map of *T. gondii* tachyzoites of RH strain and resolved over 1000 poly peptides and analyzed 71 protein spots of these proteins by MALDI-TOF MS. Among these proteins, such as dense granule antigen 1 (GRA1), GRA2, GRA7, heat-shock protein 70 (HSP70), can provide partial protection against *T. gondii* infection (Zhang, 2013). Zhou et al. (2013) investigated the proteomic profiles from differential virulent *T. gondii* strains (Types I, II, III), they showed that Type I (GT1) and Type II (PTG) have similar proteomic profiles and both are different from Type III (CTG). The contribution of differentially expressed protein in the three *T. gondii* lineages to virulence factors will be crucial to control toxoplasmosis. Similarly, the proteome analysis of *T. gondii* from bradyzoites stage and cyst stage will expand out list of potential vaccine candidates.

Neospora caninum and *T. gondii* are phylogenetically closely related Apicomplexa that share many biological, immunological, and structural features. The characterization of the cross-reactive and species-specific antigens of *N. caninum* and *T. gondii* are important in the exploration to determine the common mechanisms of parasite–host interaction; it is also useful for the selection of the cross-reactive antigens that could be used in the development of vaccines for controlling the diseases caused by these two parasites. We profiled the proteome of the *T. gondii* tachyzoite stage. Immunoblot analysis revealed that at least 31 protein spots of *T. gondii* were reacted with the anti-*T. gondii* serum, among which at least 19 spots were cross-reacted with the anti-*N. caninum* serum (Zhang, 2011). We also identified three proteins—protein disulfide isomerase (PDI), HSP70, and ribosomal protein 1 (RP1)—as crossreactive antigens between *N. caninum* and *T. gondii* by using cross-reactive monoclonal antibodies, and the antibodies from all of them could inhibit invasion of both parasites (Liao, 2005; Liao, 2006). In our previous studies, we also identified apical membrane antigen 1 (AMA1) and ribosomal phosphoprotein P0 as cross-reactive antigens between the two parasites, and the antibodies from them could inhibit the invasion or growth of both parasites (Zhang, 2007).

DNA Vaccines

DNA vaccines are based on bacterial plasmids that express the disease-specific antigen using promoter elements that are active in mammalian cells (Anderson, 2007). The antigen encoded by the plasmid is produced in host cells, either in professional antigen-presenting cells (APCs) leading to direct priming of immune responses or in non-professional cells from where the antigen can be transferred to APCs leading to cross-priming (Liu, 2005). DNA vaccines are known to induce CD4+, CD8+ T-cells and antibody responses (Liu, 2005).

The vaccine potentials of SAG1/2, HSP70/30, GRA1/2/4/6/7, ROP1/2, MIC1/2/3, M2AP, and AMA1 have also been investigated, either alone or in combination, with varying degrees of success (Makino, 2011). Vaccination with DNA vaccines encoding SAG1 gene has been found to be particularly effective in limiting mortality against both virulent and avirulent *T. gondii* challenge (Menzies, 2008).

Various efforts have been made to improve DNA vaccine potency. One main approach has been used to improve immunogenicity of DNA vaccines, that is, plasmid DNA delivery using gene gun. This technique uses gold beads that are coated with the DNA vaccines, which reduces the amount of plasmid DNA needed to induce immune responses (Anderson, 2007). Intradermal immunization by gene gun tends to target epidermal langerhans cells, which were shown to migrate rapidly to regional lymph nodes (Porgador, 1998), potentially favoring direct presentation to CD4+ and CD8+ T-cells over cross-priming (Barry, 1997). The gene gun immunization may also stimulate CTL by direct transfection of skin APC and cross-presentation (Porgador, 1998). Robust immunogenicity has been shown in many different studies using gene gun (Mohamed, 2003). Our previous works in DNA vaccines showed that gene gun immunization preferentially induces Th2-biased response, generating mostly IgG1 antibodies, and less IFN-γ, more IL-4 were produced (Yu, 2012).

Recently, heterologous prime-boost strategy has increased in popularity due to their ability to generate stronger immune responses, especially inducing a stronger immune response, compared to regimes using either a single vaccination or homologous boosting (Souza, 2005). The superiority of heterologous prime-boost is capable of inducing enhanced and persistent levels of CD8+ T-cells and Th1-type CD4+ T-cells compared to homologous boosting (Dunachie, 2003). Memory T-cells have the ability to expand rapidly upon encounter with the same antigen a second time round (Schneider, 1999). The generation of memory T-cells is at the key of numerous vaccination strategies against intracellular parasite (Reyes-Sandoval, 2007). Heterologous prime-boost immunization may generate memory T-cells (Anderson, 2007). DNA vaccines have often been used as priming vaccines in prime-boost strategy that use other vaccine modalities, such as recombinant proteins and viral vectors, to improve overall immune responses. We developed the heterologous prime-boost strategy priming with the DNA vaccine and boosting with the recombinant adenovirus as vaccination against *T. gondii* infection (Yu, 2012).

The heterologous prime-boost strategy could induce *T. gondii*-specific humoral immune responses and Th1/Th2-type immune responses. In addition, the heterologous prime-boost strategy could provide protection against *T. gondii* infection leading to an increase in survival rate and a decrease in brain cysts. In another our study, the GRA4 delivered by gene gun and attenuated vaccinia virus showed 100% survival in the heterologous prime-boost group after challenge with PLK-GFP strain. However, the vaccine failed to induce sterile immunity against tissue cysts (Zhang, 2007). Primary infection with *T. gondii* results in both humoral and cellular immune responses and confers long-term protection. This suggests that the development of an efficient vaccine is a realistic goal (Bourguin, 1993).

VIRAL VECTOR VACCINES

Recombinant viral vector may deliver the peptides to the MHC class I presentation pathway. In addition, the viral vector is capable of inducing potent, highly effective immune responses in the vaccinated hosts (Perez-Jimenez, 2006).

Furthermore, studies have shown that viral vector vaccines may indeed be used to elicit strong Th1 immune responses which are particularly useful when developing a vaccine against a disease that requires a strong Th1 protective response (Gazzinell, 1994; Campos-Neto, 2005). Viral delivery of immunogenic antigens has been tested against *T. gondii*. Viruses may provide an entryway into the host cell cytoplasm or nucleus, allowing native organelles to express the encoded *T. gondii* proteins (Srivastava, 2003). These foreign antigens enter the MHC class I presentation pathway. When an appropriate peptide/MHC complex is present on the cell surface, complex activates CD8+ T-cells. CD8+ T-cells in turn are able to destroy parasites in cells, either through direct cytolysis or through the secretion of IFN-γ, leading to the production of nitric oxide and parasite death (Srivastava, 2003). Viral vectors also induced an IgG antibody response, and specific CD4+ T-cells through cross-priming (Jooss, 2003). Multiple viral vectors are available that are considered safe and are being tested in animals. Poxviruses, adenoviruses, herpesviruses, influenza viruses, pseudorabies virus and baculoviruses have been used to construct viral vectors for protection against *T. gondii* infection.

Modified vaccinia ankara (MVA) cannot replicate in mammalian cells and is non-pathogenic (Paoletti, 1996). MVA vector expressing ROP2 could induce specific antibody, and delay the time of death after challenge with 300 RH strain tachyzoites, while vaccination with MVA-ROP2 failed to reduce brain cysts when mice were orally challenged with 20 ME49 cysts (Roque-Resendiz, 2004).

Replication-defective, E1-E3 gene deleted adenovirus vectors must be grown in a packaging cell line, such as human embryonic kidney (HEK) 293 cells, which express the E1-E3 proteins (He, 1998). Replicaction-defective adenovirus is not able to replicate in other cells (Limbach, 2009). For these reasons, adenovirus-based vaccines have been developed for humans and animals (McCoy, 2007; Limbach, 2009). A study recently reported preliminary studies with three recombinant adenoviruses, expressing SAG1, SAG2, or SAG3 (Caetano, 2006).

Immunization of BALB/c mice with these viruses induced both antibodies and IFN-γ responses. However, upon challenge with a lethal dose of RH strain these mice were not protected. Conversely, challenge with a P-Br strain did show a reduction of tissue cysts burden by 80% in the brain (Caetano, 2006). And then, this research team tested the three different viruses in the highly susceptible C57BL/6 mice. They verified that only AdSAG1, but neither

AdSAG2 nor AdSAG3, induces protective immunity in the highly susceptible C57BL/6 mice orally challenged with 10 cysts of ME49 strain. The critical role of Myeloid Differentiation Factor 88 (MyD88), IL-12, IFN-γ and CD8+ T cells in the anti-*Toxoplasma* protective immunity are elicited by AdSAG1 (Mendes, 2011).

A feline herpesvirus type 1 (FHV1) has been selected as carrier because it spreads among cats contagiously, thereby hopefully disseminating the vaccine to neighboring domestic and stray cats (Mishima, 2002). FHV1 expressing ROP2 induced specific antibodies, and reduced brain tissue cysts in cats, but did not reduce oocyst secretion.

The baculovirus *Autographa californica* multiple nucleopolyhedrosis virus (AcMNPV) is enveloped, double-stranded DNA virus that naturally infect insects. To enable expression of a recombinant protein in mammalian cells a promoter active in the target cells, such as CMV (cytomegalovirus), RSV (rous sarcoma virus), or CAG (chichen β-actin promoter) must be used because *polh* is inactive in these cells. Hofmann et al. (1995) showed for the first time that recombinant AcMNPV that contains the CMV promoter is able to transducer human hepatocytes and drive expression of luciferase reporter gene under the control of this promoter. These attributes have sparked explosive interests to develop baculovirus as a vector vaccine candidate, in which the antigen can be expressed by the vector within the host cells. The immunization of a VSVG-pseudotyped baculovirus expressing SAG1 triggered IFN-γ production and 50% survival was obtained in mice challenged with RH strain (Fang, 2010).

Pseudorabies virus (PRV) has been shown to be an excellent vector for expression and delivery of foreign antigen (van Zijl, 1991). A prime-boost vaccination with DNA vaccine pVAX-SAG1 and recombinant pseudorabies virus rPRV-SAG1 showed an increased survival time (Shang, 2009). A cocktail vaccine using rPRV-SAG1 and rPRV-MIC3 was tested in mice challenged with *T. gondii*. The cocktail vaccine elicited humoral and Th1 cellular immune response and increased survival time (Nie, 2011).

The heterologous prime-boost strategy has been tested using different viral vectors. Machado et al. showed that mice primed with a recombinant influenza virus and boosted with recombinant adenovirus encoding SAG2 displayed significant reduction of parasite burden after challenge with the P-Br strain of *T. gondii*. However, the significant protection cannot be achieved after a single immunization (Machado, 2010). The heterologous prime-boost strategy was considered useful method to control *T. gondii* infection.

LIVE PROTOZOAN VECTOR VACCINES

Since *T. gondii* is an intracellular parasite, strategy with avirulent parasite against virulent parasite has been evaluated. As mentioned in the previous section, *N. caninum* is an apicomplexan parasite that is morphologically very similar to *T. gondii* (Lindsay, 1993). *N. caninum* is an important cause of bovine abortion (Nietfeld, 1992) and neurological disease in dogs (Dubey, 1988). There is no evidence that *N. caninum* can infect or cause disease in humans (Graham, 1999). Therefore, the virulence-associated gene knockout parasites will be desirable for developing a safe, attenuated *N. caninum* vector vaccine to control toxoplasmosis in animals. *N. caninum* has been shown that cellular and humoral responses were induced following experimental infection by *N. caninum* tachyzoites or oocysts in both non-pregnant and pregnant animals (De Marez, 1999). Especially, a T cell immune response could be induced by *N. caninum* in an infected host, which is at least partially mediated by IL-12 and IFN-γ (Andrianarivo, 2001). Likewise, host resistance to *T. gondii* is highly dependent on the early production of IL-12 as well as IFN-γ by both CD4+ and CD8+ T cells. It has also been reported that mice infected with *N. caninum* were protected against a lethal challenge infection with *T. gondii* (Kasper, 1995). The immunity produced by *N. caninum* raised interest in its use as a vaccine vector against toxoplasmosis, a disease whose control is prominently dependent on T cell activity. Howe et al. (1997) has documented that *N. caninum* is a suitable vector to express the genes from *T. gondii* as native forms. Zhang et al. (2010) recently reported preliminary studies with *N. caninum* expressing TgSAG1. In this study, Nc/TgSAG1 could induce TgSAG1-specific Th1-dominant immune responses associated with IFN-γ in a mouse model. Immunization of BALB/c mice with Nc/TgSAG1 showed 83.33% survived after a lethal-dose challenge infection with 500 *T. gondii* Beverley strain. Live protozoal parasite vaccines have opened up a promising approach against toxoplasmosis.

CURRENT TRENDS OF VACCINE DEVELOPMENT AGAINST *TOXOPLASMA GONDII* INFECTION

Future strategies to design new vaccines for *T. gondii* should be considered to search virulence-associated molecules by using genomics, transcriptomics, and proteomics approaches and create attenuated live vaccines by disrupting virulent genes. For example, a promising vaccine mutant has been generated with a disruption of carbamoyl phosphate synthetase II (CPSII) (Fox, 2002). In the absence of uracil, CPSII knockout *T. gondii* invaded host cells normally but failed to replicate. CPSII knockout parasites did not kill BALB/c mice, and mice infected with CPSII knockout parasites 40 days previously were resistant to a lethal challenge with 200 RH strain tachyzoites (Fox, 2002).

REFERENCES

Ferguson, D.J.P., Dubremetz, J.F. (2007). *The ultrastructure of Toxoplasma gondii.* Tokyo: Academic Press, Elsevier, p.19-46.

Roberts, C.W., Gazzinelli, R.T. (2007). *Adaptive immunity and genetics of the host immune response.* Tokyo: Academic Press, Elsevier, p.609-697.

Anderson, R.J., Schneider, J. (2007). Plasmid DNA and viral vector-based vaccines for the treatment of cancer. *Vaccine* 25 Suppl 2:B24-34.

Andrianarivo, A.G., Barr, B.C. (2001). Immune responses in pregnant cattle and bovine fetuses following experimental infection with *Neospora caninum. Parasitol. Res.* 87:817-25.

Barry, M.A., Johnston, S.A. (1997). Biological features of genetic immunization. *Vaccine* 15:788-91.

Belli, S.I., Walker, R.A. (2005). Global protein expression analysis in apicomplexan parasites: current status. *Proteomics* 5:918-24.

Bourguin, I., Chardes, T. (1993). Oral immunization with *Toxoplasma gondii* antigens in association with cholera toxin induces enhanced protective and cell-mediated immunity in C57BL/6 mice. *Infect. Immun.* 61:2082-8.

Brown, C.R., David,C.S. (1994). Effects of human class I transgenes on *Toxoplasma gondii* cyst formation. *J. Immunol.* 152:4537-41.

Buzoni-Gatel, D., Schulthess, J. (2006). Mucosal defences against orally acquired protozoan parasites, emphasis on *Toxoplasma gondii* infections. *Cell Microbiol.* 8:535-44.

Caetano, B.C., Bruna-Romero, O. (2006). Vaccination with replication-deficient recombinant adenoviruses encoding the main surface antigens of *toxoplasma gondii* induces immune response and protection against infection in mice. *Hum. Gene Ther.* 17:415-26.

Campos-Neto, A. (2005). What about Th1/Th2 in cutaneous leishmaniasis vaccine discovery? *Braz. J. Med. Biol. Res.* 38:979-84.

Casadevall, A., Pirofski, L.A. (2006). A reappraisal of humoral immunity based on mechanisms of antibody-mediated protection against intracellular pathogens. *Adv. Immunol.* 91:1-44.

Channon, J.Y., Seguin, R.M. (2000). Differential infectivity and division of *Toxoplasma gondii* in human peripheral blood leukocytes. *Infect. Immun.* 68: 4822-6.

Cohen, A.M., Rumpel, K. (2002). Characterisation of global protein expression by two-dimensional electrophoresis and mass spectrometry: proteomics of *Toxoplasma gondii. Int. J. Parasitol.* 32:39-51.

Courret, N., Darche, S. (2006). CD11c- and CD11b-expressing mouse leukocytes transport single Toxoplasma gondii tachyzoites to the brain. *Blood* 107:309-16.

De Marez, T., Liddell, S. (1999). Oral infection of calves with *Neospora caninum* oocysts from dogs: humoral and cellular immune responses. *Int J Parasitol* 29:1647-57.

Dubey, J.P. (2004). Toxoplasmosis-a waterborne zoonosis. *Vet. Parasitol.* 126: 57-72.

Dubey, J.P., Carpenter,J.L. (1988). Newly recognized fatal protozoan disease of dogs. *J. Am. Vet. Med. Assoc.* 192:1269-85.

Dubey, J.P., Jones, J.L. (2008). *Toxoplasma gondii* infection in humans and animals in the United States. *Int. J. Parasitol.* 38:1257-78.

Dunachie, S.J., Hill, A.V. (2003). Prime-boost strategies for malaria vaccine development. *J. Exp. Biol.* 206:3771-9.

Fang, R., Feng, H. (2010). Construction and immunogenicity of pseudotype baculovirus expressing *Toxoplasma gondii* SAG1 protein in BALB/c mice model. *Vaccine* 28:1803-7.

Fox, B.A., Bzik D.J. (2002). De novo pyrimidine biosynthesis is required for virulence of *Toxoplasma gondii. Nature* 415:926-9.

Frenkel, J.K., Taylor, D.W. (1982). Toxoplasmosis in immunoglobulin M-suppressed mice. *Infect. Immun.* 38:360-7.

Gazzinelli, R.T., Wysocka, M. (1994). Parasite-induced IL-12 stimulates early IFN-gamma synthesis and resistance during acute infection with *Toxoplasma gondii. J. Immunol.* 153:2533-43.

Gazzinelli, R., Xu, Y. (1992). Simultaneous depletion of CD4+ and CD8+ T lymphocytes is required to reactivate chronic infection with *Toxoplasma gondii. J. Immunol.* 149:175-80.

Graham, D.A., Calvert, V. (1999). Absence of serological evidence for human *Neospora caninum* infection. *Vet. Rec.* 144:672-3.

He, T.C., Zhou, S. (1998). A simplified system for generating recombinant adenoviruses. *Proc. Natl. Acad. Sci. USA* 95:2509-14.

Hofmann, C., Sandig, V. (1995). Efficient gene transfer into human hepatocytes by baculovirus vectors. *Proc. Natl. Acad. Sci. USA* 92:10099-103.

Howe, D.K., Mercier, C. (1997). Expression of Toxoplasma gondii genes in the closely-related apicomplexan parasite *Neospora caninum. Mol. Biochem. Parasitol.* 86:29-36.

Innes, E.A., Bartley, P.M. (2009). Veterinary vaccines against *Toxoplasma gondii. Mem. Inst. Oswaldo Cruz* 104:246-51.

Innes, E.A., Vermeulen, A.N. (2006). Vaccination as a control strategy against the coccidial parasites Eimeria, *Toxoplasma* and *Neospora. Parasitology* 133 Suppl:S145-68.

Johnson, L.L., Sayles, P. C. (2002). Deficient humoral responses underlie susceptibility to *Toxoplasma gondii* in CD4-deficient mice. *Infect. Immun.* 70:185-91.

Jones, J.L., and Dubey, J.P. (2012). Foodborne toxoplasmosis. *Clin. Infect. Dis.* 55:845-51.

Jongert, E., Roberts, C.W. (2009). Vaccines against *Toxoplasma gondii*: challenges and opportunities. *Mem. Inst. Oswaldo Cruz* 104:252-66.

Jooss, K., Chirmule, N. (2003). Immunity to adenovirus and adeno-associated viral vectors: implications for gene therapy. *Gene. Ther.* 10:955-63.

Kang, H., Remington, J.S. (2000). Decreased resistance of B cell-deficient mice to infection with *Toxoplasma gondii* despite unimpaired expression of IFN-gamma, TNF-alpha, and inducible nitric oxide synthase. *J. Immunol.* 164:2629-34.

Kasper, L.H., Matsuura, T. (1995). IL-7 stimulates protective immunity in mice against the intracellular pathogen, *Toxoplasma gondii. J. Immunol.* 155: 4798-804.

Klade, C.S. (2002). Proteomics approaches towards antigen discovery and vaccine development. *Curr. Opin. Mol. Ther.* 4:216-23.

Liao, M., Ma, L. (2006). Identification of a protein disulfide isomerase of *Neospora caninum* in excretory-secretory products and its IgA binding and enzymatic activities. *Vet. Parasitol.* 139:47-56.

Liao, M., Xuan, X. (2005). Identification and characterization of cross-reactive antigens from *Neospora caninum* and *Toxoplasma gondii. Parasitology* 130:481-8.

Limbach, K.J., Richie, T.L. (2009). Viral vectors in malaria vaccine development. *Parasite Immunol.* 31:501-19.

Lindsay, D.S., Speer, C.A. (1993). Use of infected cultured cells to compare ultrastructural features of *Neospora caninum* from dogs and *Toxoplasma gondii*. *Am. J. Vet. Res.* 54:103-6.

Liu, M.A., Ulmer J.B. (2005). Human clinical trials of plasmid DNA vaccines. *Adv. Genet.* 55:25-40.

Machado, A.V., Caetano,B.C. (2010). Prime and boost immunization with influenza and adenovirus encoding the *Toxoplasma gondii* surface antigen 2 (SAG2) induces strong protective immunity. *Vaccine* 28:3247-56.

Makino, M., Uemura, N. (2011). Innate immunity in DNA vaccine with *Toxoplasma gondii*-heat shock protein 70 gene that induces DC activation and Th1 polarization. *Vaccine* 29:1899-905.

McCoy, K., Tatsis, N. (2007). Effect of preexisting immunity to adenovirus human serotype 5 antigens on the immune responses of nonhuman primates to vaccine regimens based on human- or chimpanzee-derived adenovirus vectors. *J Virol* 81:6594-604.

Mendes, E.A., Caetano, B.C. (2011). MyD88-dependent protective immunity elicited by adenovirus 5 expressing the surface antigen 1 from *Toxoplasma gondii* is mediated by CD8(+) T lymphocytes. *Vaccine* 29: 4476-84.

Menzies, F.M., Henriquez, F.L. (2008). Immunological control of congenital toxoplasmosis in the murine model. *Immunol. Lett.* 115:83-9.

Mishima, M., Xuan, X. (2002). Recombinant feline herpesvirus type 1 expressing *Toxoplasma gondi* ROP2 antigen inducible protective immunity in cats. *Parasitol. Res.* 88:144-9.

Mohamed, R.M., Aosai, F. (2003). Induction of protective immunity by DNA vaccination with *Toxoplasma gondii* HSP70, HSP30 and SAG1 genes. *Vaccine* 21:2852-61.

Montoya, J.G., Liesenfeld, O. (2004). Toxoplasmosis. *Lancet* 363:1965-76.

Neyer, L.E., Grunig,G. (1997). Role of interleukin-10 in regulation of T-cell-dependent and T-cell-independent mechanisms of resistance to *Toxoplasma gondii*. *Infect. Immun.* 65:1675-82.

Nie, H., Fang, R. (2011). Immunogenicity and protective efficacy of two recombinant pseudorabies viruses expressing *Toxoplasma gondii* SAG1 and MIC3 proteins. *Vet. Parasitol.* 181:215-21.

Nietfeld, J.C., Dubey, J.P. (1992). Neospora-like protozoan infection as a cause of abortion in dairy cattle. *J. Vet. Diagn. Invest.* 4:223-6.

Paoletti, E. (1996). Applications of pox virus vectors to vaccination: an update. *Proc. Natl. Acad. Sci. USA* 93:11349-53.

Perez-Jimenez, E., Kochan,G. (2006). MVA-LACK as a safe and efficient vector for vaccination against leishmaniasis. *Microbes Infect.* 8:810-22.
Porgador, A., Irvine, K.R. (1998). Predominant role for directly transfected dendritic cells in antigen presentation to CD8+ T cells after gene gun immunization. *J. Exp. Med.* 188:1075-82.
Reyes-Sandoval, A., Harty, J.T. (2007). Viral vector vaccines make memory T cells against malaria. *Immunology* 121:158-65.
Roque-Resendiz, J.L., Rosales, R. (2004). MVA ROP2 vaccinia virus recombinant as a vaccine candidate for toxoplasmosis. *Parasitology* 128: 397-405.
Sayles, P.C., Gibson, G.W. (2000). B cells are essential for vaccination-induced resistance to virulent Toxoplasma gondii. *Infect. Immun.* 68:1026-33.
Scharton-Kersten, T.M., Yap, G.J. (1997). Inducible nitric oxide is essential for host control of persistent but not acute infection with the intracellular pathogen *Toxoplasma gondii. J. Exp. Med.* 185:1261-73.
Schneider, J., Gilbert, S.C. (1999). Induction of CD8+ T cells using heterologous prime-boost immunisation strategies. *Immunol. Rev.* 170: 29-38.
Shang, L., Liu, Q. (2009). Protection in mice immunized with a heterologous prime-boost regime using DNA and recombinant pseudorabies expressing TgSAG1 against *Toxoplasma gondii* challenge. *Vaccine* 27:2741-5.
Souza, A.P., Haut,L. (2005). Recombinant viruses as vaccines against viral diseases. *Braz. J. Med. Biol. Res.* 38:509-22.
Srivastava, I.K., Liu, M.A. (2003). Gene vaccines. *Ann. Intern. Med.* 138: 550-9.
Tenter, A.M., Heckeroth, A.R. (2000). *Toxoplasma gondii*: from animals to humans. *Int. J. Parasitol.* 30:1217-58.
van Zijl, M., Wensvoort, G. (1991). Live attenuated pseudorabies virus expressing envelope glycoprotein E1 of hog cholera virus protects swine against both pseudorabies and hog cholera. *J. Virol.* 65:2761-5.
Weiss, L.M., Kim, K. (2000). The development and biology of bradyzoites of *Toxoplasma gondii. Front. Biosci.* 5:D391-405.
Wilkins, M.F., O'Connell, E. (1988). Toxoplasmosis in sheep III. Further evaluation of the ability of a live *Toxoplasma gondii* vaccine to prevent lamb losses and reduce congenital infection following experimental oral challenge. *N. Z .Vet. J.* 36:86-9.
Yu, L., Yamagishi, J. (2012). Protective effect of a prime-boost strategy with plasmid DNA followed by recombinant adenovirus expressing TgAMA1

as vaccines against *Toxoplasma gondii* infection in mice. *Parasitol. Int.* 61: 481-6.

Zhang, G., Huang, X. (2010). Construction of Neospora caninum stably expressing TgSAG1 and evaluation of its protective effects against *Toxoplasma gondii* infection in mice. *Vaccine* 28:7243-7.

Zhang, G., Huong,V.T. (2007). A heterologous prime-boost vaccination regime using DNA and a vaccinia virus, both expressing GRA4, induced protective immunity against *Toxoplasma gondii* infection in mice. *Parasitology* 134:1339-46.

Zhang, H., Compaore, M.K. (2007). Apical membrane antigen 1 is a cross-reactive antigen between *Neospora caninum* and *Toxoplasma gondii*, and the anti-NcAMA1 antibody inhibits host cell invasion by both parasites. *Mol. Biochem. Parasitol.* 151:205-12.

Zhang, H., Lee, E.G. (2011). Identification of the cross-reactive and species-specific antigens between *Neospora caninum* and *Toxoplasma gondii* tachyzoites by a proteomics approach. *Parasitol. Res.* 109:899-911.

Zhang, N., Chen, J. (2013). Vaccines against *Toxoplasma gondii*: new developments and perspectives. *Expert. Rev. Vaccines.* 12:1287-99.

Zhou, H., Zhao, Q. (2013). Differential proteomic profiles from distinct *Toxoplasma gondii* strains revealed by 2D-difference gel electrophoresis. *Exp. Parasitol.* 133:376-382.

In: Recent Advances in Toxoplasmosis Research ISBN: 978-1-63117-914-3
Editor: Connor M. Lee

Chapter 9

MOLECULAR DIAGNOSIS IN TOXOPLASMOSIS

I. B. Hernandez-Cortazar[1], K. Y. Acosta-Viana[1], E. Guzman-Marín[1], A. Ortega-Pacheco[1] and M. Jiménez-Coello[1]

[1]Universidad Autonoma de Yucatan, Mexico

ABSTRACT

Toxoplasmosis is a worldwide parasite disease caused by the aplicomplexa *Toxoplasma gondii.* This important parasitic infection remains persistently in infected individuals and may affect to both humans and animals. The diagnosis of toxoplasmosis has always been a challenge. Serology has been an usual tool for the detection of infection. However, given that toxoplasmosis is of great clinical relevance in pregnant women and immunosuppressed patients, there is always an increasing interest in developing alternatives for timely diagnosis to determine the presence and levels of parasitemia. The molecular diagnostic tools of *T. gondii* include the Polymerase Chain Reaction (PCR) with its variants, such as end-point PCR, real time PCR, and lamp, which permit a very specific determination of the genome of the protozoa from different biological samples. For this purpose PCR from amniotic fluid, placental and brain tissues, whole blood, cerebrospinal fluid, urine, vitreous fluid, aqueous humor, bronchoalveolar lavage fluid and pleural and peritoneal fluids has proved of value to diagnose *T.gondii*. The most common use of PCR is for prenatal diagnosis of the congenital infection using amniotic fluid samples. Several factor may influence the success of molecular detection of *T.gondii* such as the method of purification of DNA samples and very specific technical details that determine the sensitivity and specificity of diagnostic tests, such as the selection of primers, the use of hot start, the use of the enzyme uracyl-DNA-glycosylase to prevent carryover contamination, the size of the PCR product and use of internal control or nested PCR.

The aim of this chapter is to point out and discuss the current and more successful molecular biology techniques for the diagnosis and quantification of *Toxoplasma gondii* in clinical samples.

1. Introduction to Toxoplasmosis

Toxoplasmosis is a parasitic zoonosis of major importance since it is spread throughout the world. Felines, particularly domestic cats have special importance in the epidemiology of the disease because they carried out the sexual and asexual reproduction phase of the parasite and make them able to excrete infective oocysts in their feces (Dubey, 1995; Kravetz et al., 2005). This parasite affects most mammals (including humans) and birds, which are intermediate hosts. Farm animal species are especially important in the epidemiology of the disease because they intended for human consumption (Dubey, 1996; Martinez et al., 1998; Tenter, 2001). Several intermediate hosts can become infected by ingesting sporulated oocysts from contaminated soil and water; by ingesting raw meat containing tissue cysts or by vertical transmission. Other methods of infection occur less often by blood or leukocyte transfusions or by organ transplants (Kravetz, 2005; Martino and Bretange, 2005).

It is important to differentiate the infection phase with toxoplasmosis disease because infections occur at different stages such as acute clinical, sub-clinical or asymptomatic forms (Saadatnia and Golkar, 2012; Dubey et al., 1997) with cycles of reinfection or reactivation.

1.1. Diagnosis of Toxoplasmosis

Diagnosis of Toxoplasmosis has been intended by isolation, histological, serological and molecular methods or by their combination (Dubey et al., 2009). The isolation of *T. gondii* can be accomplished from tissue culture or from laboratory animals (Dehkordi et al., 2013; Pardini et al., 2013). The parasite can be isolated from patients by *in vitro* or *in vivo* methods; the choice of specimen used as inoculum will depend on the circumstances, but secretions, fluids (i.e. cerebrospinal) or tissue collected by biopsy (lymph nodes, base of the tongue or brain tissue) are very good options where the parasite can be founded (Al Qassab et al., 2009; Dubey et al., 2009).

Serological methods are widely implemented and are based on finding the presence of anti-*T.gondii* antibodies in patient sera using immuno biological methods. There are many serological techniques available, (i.e. Sabin-Fieldman dye test, the indirect hemagglutination assay, the indirect fluorescence antibody assay and the inmmunosorbent agglutination assay test within others) (Edvinsson, 2006).

In immunocompetent adults, the presence of specific antibodies (sero conversion) against *T. gondii* only indicates a previous contact between the patient and the parasite. The use of indirect ELISA technique is widely used to perform the serological diagnosis and can detect both the presence/absence of specific antibodies and can also allows a semi-quantitative estimate, which can give an idea of the antibody concentration (IU per mL of serum). The ELISA assay is one of the most widely used methodologies for the detection of IgM and IgG antibodies including *T. gondii*. The presence of anti-*Toxoplasma gondii* IgM can be detected soon after infection whereas IgG could be measurable after 7 to 14 days post-infection and may have lifelong persistence. However, it has been also described that IgM remains present and can be detected for a long time. With the purpose to differentiate a recent from an older infection, the affinity test has been used; the binding force of antibodies is usually lower for IgG, generated shortly after a primary infection and increase over the time. With this modification, an ELISA test measuring also avidity can be used to discriminate a recently acquired infection from an infection acquired over 6 months ago (Lopez-Mori et al., 2013; Baquero-Artigao et al., 2013; Villard et al., 2013).

The use of molecular biology is very useful to complement all other diagnostic alternatives for *T. gondii*. The molecular techniques have a high sensitivity and specificity. However, some of the limitations are the need to be performed by trained personnel, the need of good quality samples under aseptic conditions, the need to be carried out in appropriate facilities, the time needed to obtained results, and their relatively expensive cost. Their greatest contribution nevertheless is that it can accurately determine the presence of DNA of the parasite in the analyzed samples in a relatively short period of time (compared to *in vitro* or *in vivo* like isolation in cell culture or in rodents), which is of great importance at the time of taking decision when assessing the patient's condition.

There are a lot of reports and research studies in both humans and animals, where different molecular biology methodologies have been used to detect the presence of *T. gondii* DNA; much of these reports are predominantly based on the PCR technique (i.e. endpoint PCR, real time PCR, nested PCR, Lamp PCR, etc.). More recently Texeira et al., (2013) compared four different molecular methodologies and concluded than real time PCR is the best option for detection (at least in amniotic fluid samples) of congenital toxoplasmosis.

Molecular diagnostics of toxoplasmosis is generally based on the detection of a specific DNA sequence, using different assays and protocols, mostly from highly conserved regions such as the B1 gene repeated 35 times in the genome, 529 bp repetitive element with about 200-300 copies in the genome but it is not present in all the *T. gondii* strains, ITS-1 (internal transcribed spacer) that exists in 110 copies and 18S rDNA gene sequences (Table 1). Qualitative PCR protocols for the detection of single copy genes such as the P30 gene appeared less sensitive and they are rarely used for diagnostic purposes (Jones et al., 2000; Ivović et al., 2012).

In this chapter some of these reports and strategies used for detection (and in some cases quantification) of B1 gene of the parasite DNA in biological samples are described from both human and animal patients.

Table 1. *Toxoplasma gondii* DNA detection markers (Ivović et al., 2012)

Markers	No. of copies	Reference
B1	~35	Wahab et al., 2010 Correia et al., 2010 Okay et al., 2009
529 pb (AF146527)	200-300	da Silva RC et al., 2011 Yera et al., 2009 Vujanić et al., 2011
ITS -1 or 18S rDNA	~ 110	Truppel et al., 2010 Miller et al., 2004
P30	Single copy gene	Buchbinder et al., 2003 Eida et al., 2009 Cardona et al., 2009

We also describe some of the methodologies standardized by this research group to efficiently detect the presence of the parasite and its concentration in different types of biological samples from humans and various domestic animal species, using the basic material and equipment of molecular biology.

Molecular Detection of T. gondii in Humans

Despite the existence of different sets of primers for different DNA targets (Weiss, 1995), the results obtained can be very variable, so a general consensus of the best protocols may be difficult to achieve. However, it is possible to distinguish most successful options to improve *T. gondii* DNA detection. Different amplification targets have been researched to detect the presence of the DNA of the parasite including the located in the genes: B1, 18S, P30, or 529 bp repeat element (and others like SAG2, SAG3, GRA4 and ROP1), but different results have been reported depending mostly on the target used and the clinical sample evaluated.

Studies aimed to detect targets located in the B1 gen have been those that have shown greater efficiency and sensitivity, because this is a gene highly repeated in the genome of the parasite (35 fold-repetitive element present in all the *T. gondii* strains) and thus increasing the likelihood of detection. Some of the most representative reports detecting *T. gondii* DNA using end point PCR, nested PCR, LAMP PCR and Real time PCR are cited in table 2.

These studies can detect efficiently the parasite DNA in different clinical samples, including amniotic fluid, cerebral spinal fluid (CFS), brain tissue (fixated or paraffin included), peripheral blood, aqueous humor, placenta and others.

All these clinical samples could be successfully used for *T. gondii* detection if is chosen an appropriated DNA extraction technique. Protocols based in adsorcion - desorcion (ie. through chromatography columns) could be excellent options because are quick and allows to obtain a good quality and amount of DNA material for evaluation. However, for samples in liquid form, is recommended to concentrate them at least in 1 mL (for CFS or peripheral blood) (Alfonso et al., 2013, Jalal 2004) to increase the probability to detect the agent.

On other hand, the diagnosis with a modification of the PCR technique like nested PCR or semi-nested PCR have been also widely reported. It is important to comment that with a double round of amplification, the probability of detection is highly increased, but with the risk o a false positive result, due the manipulation of the template for the preparation of second round of reaction.

For that reason, if these strategy for *T. gondii* DNA detection is selected, the implementation and preparation of every round of reactions must be carefully done, and performed by experienced personal. Some authors have suggested that nested PCR or seminested PCR could be good options for detection in laboratories where a real time PCR equipment is not available (Alfonso et al., 2013).

Finally, the use of Real Time PCR, facilitate the diagnosis of *T. gondii* in clinical laboratories. These variant of PCR allows not only detecting the presence of DNA of the parasite, but also provides quantitative information about the amplification target in a quick way.

Molecular Detection of T. gondii in Animals

For the detection of *T. gondii* DNA from domestic or wild animals different strategies have been described. The molecular detection using PCR and its variants have been successfully used (Table 3).

The most frequent amplification targets used amplify B1 gene. Due to the rol of different animal species as definite hosts or reservoirs, domestic and wild animals play a relevant role in the transmission, persistence and risk of infection to humans (particularly through the consumption of the infected animals meat).

For those reasons, there is a special interest in detecting DNA of the parasite for clinical diagnosis as well as for meat monitoring, to determine the presence and amount of the parasite and consequently to improve the production systems of innocuous meat as well reduce the risk of human infections.

An important aspect to consider when molecular approaches are used in the detection of *T. gondii* DNA detection is the type of clinical sample to evaluate. The most reported samples include blood, tissue (mainly brain, tongue, heart and spleen), placenta, aborted material, and less commonly CFS and aqueous humor.

Due to importance in public health, several authors have reported different strategies of PCR (end Point, nested or qPCR) to detect the presence of *T. gondii* DNA from feline stool samples (Dubey et al., 2009; Mancianti et al., 2010; Salant et al., 2010; Berger-Schoch et al., 2012; Lalonde and Gajadhar, 2012). These methodologies can be useful for both clinical evaluation of a feline or environmental monitoring (ie. sampling in parks, gardens, etc.).

Table 2. Representative PCR methods based in the amplification of B1 gen of *Toxoplasma* in biological samples from humans

Format PCR and detection	Target gene	Primer and probe sequences	Sample	Study population	Reference
Real-time quantitative PCR Nested PCR	B1	F: TOXO-F: TCCCCTCTGCTGGCGAAAAGT R: TOXO-R: AGCGTTCGTGGTCAACTATCGATTG TaqMan probe: 6FAM-TCTGTGCAACTTTGGTGTATTCGCAG-TAMRA Fo: TOXO 1: GGAACTGCATCCGTTCATGAG Ro: TOXO 2: TCTTTAAAGCGTTCGTGGTC Fi: TOXO 4: TGCATAGGTTGCAGTCACTG Ri: TOXO 2: TCTTTAAAGCGTTCGTGGTC	Paraffin-embedded fetal tissue sections	Fetuses	Lin et al., 2000
Conventional PCR Nested PCR Nested PCR	B1	F: B22: TGTTCTGTCCTATCGCAACG R: B23: TGGGTCTACGTCGATGGCATGACAAC Fo: S1: TGTTCTGTCCTATCGCAACG Ro: AS1: ACGGATGCAGTTCCTTTCTG Fi: S2: TCTTCCCAGACGTGGATTTC Ri: AS2: CTCGACAATACGCTGCTTGA Fo: T1: GGAACTGCATCCGTTCATGAG Ro: T4: GGCGACCAATCTGCGAATACACC Fi: T2: TGCATAGGTTGCAGTCACTG Ri: T3: TCTTTAAAGCGTTCGGGTC	CSF (cerebrospinal fluid)	AIDS patients	Alfonso et al., 2013

Table 2. (Continued)

Format PCR and detection	Target gene	Primer and probe sequences	Sample	Study population	Reference
Conventional PCR	B1	F: B22: TGTTCTGTCCTATCGCAACG R: B23: TGGGTCTACGTCGATGGCATGACAAC F: T1: GGAACTGCATCCGTTCATGAG R: T2: TGCATAGGTTGCAGTCACTG	AF, placenta, cord blood, peripheral blood	Women with suspicion of toxoplasmosis	Chabbert et al., 2004
Real-time quantitative PCR	B1	F: TX2F: CTAGTATCGTGCGGCAATGTG R: TX2R: GGCAGCGTCTCTTCCTCTTTT TaqMan probe: TX2M1: FAM-CCACCTCGCCTCTTGG(NFQ-MGB)	Peripheral blood	Individuals with suspicion of acute or chronic toxoplasmosis	Kompalic-Cristo et al., 2007
Conventional PCR Real-time quantitative PCR	B1	F: B22: AACGGGCGAGTAGCACCTGAGGAGA R: B23: TGGGTCTACGTCGATGGCATGACAAC F: B1Tg-F: CAAGCAGCGTATTGTCGAGTAGAT-39 R: B1Tg-R: GCGTCTCTTTCATTCCCACATTTT Probe TaqMan: B1Tg-TM: FAM-CAGAAAGGAACTGCATCCGTT	CSF and blood	Patients suspected of cerebral toxoplasmosis	Mesquita et al., 2010
Real-time quantitative PCR	B1	F: Primer F-TCCCCTCTGCTGGCGAAAAGT R: Primer R-AGCGTTCGTGGTCAACTATCGATTG TaqMan Probe: 6FAM-TCTGTGCAACTTTGGTGTATTCGCAG	Ocular fluid	Patients with clinically suspected ocular toxoplasmosis	Sugita et al., 2011

Format PCR and detection	Target gene	Primer and probe sequences	Sample	Study population	Reference
Nested PCR	B1	Fo: P3: CTTCAAGCAGCGTATTGTCG Ro: P7b: TCTTTAAAGCGTTCGTGGTC Fi: P7: TAAAGCGTTCGTGGTCAACT Ri: P8: GGAACTGCATCCGTTCATGA	Blood	Allogenic stem cell recipients	Hierl et al., 2004
Nested-PCR	B1	Fo: TCAAGCAGCGTATTGTCGAG Ro: CCGCAGCGACTTCTATCTCT Fi: GGAACTGCATCCGTTCATGAG Ri: TCTTTAAAGCGTTCGTGGTC	Blood samples	Children whit cancer Liver transplant recipients	Fallahi et al., 2014 Caner et al., 2008
Semi-Nested PCR	B1	F: GAACTGCATCCGTTCATG R: TCTTTAAAGCGTTCGTGGTC	Paraffin-embedded blocks of aborted placenta	Spontaneous Aborted Fetuses	Asgari et al., 2013
Nested-PCR	B1	Fo: GGAACTGCATCCGTTCATGAG Ro: TCTTTAAAGCGTTCGTGGTC Ri: TGCATAGGTTGCAGTCACTG Ri: GGCGACCAATCTGCGAATACACC	Aqueous humor	Patient with postoperative fibrinous uveitis	Jones et al., 2000
LAMP	B1	B3: ACGTGACAGTGAAGAGAGGA F3: CAGATGTGCTAAAGGCGTCA BIP: TGTTCGCTGTCTGTCTAGGGCAGGTGGTCGACTTCATGGGA FIP: AGGCGGAACCAACGGAAATCCTTGCTGTTCTGTCCTATCGC	Blood CSF	Patients with active toxoplasmosis Patients with suspected toxoplasmic encephalitis	Lau et al., 2010 Mikita et al., 2013

Table 3. Targets for specific detection of *Toxoplasma gondii* by PCR in animals

Format PCR	Target gene	Primer and probe sequences	Sample	Species	Reference
Real-Time PCR	B1	F: GGAGGACTGGCAACCTGGTGTCG R: TTGTTTCACCCGGACCGTTTAGCAG	Diaphragm tissue	Pigs, Cattle and sheep	Berger-Schoch et al., 2011
Heminested-PCR	B1	B1a GAGAGGTCCGCCCCCACAAC B1b CTGCTGGTGCGAGGGGAGTG B1c CAGGAGTTGGATTTTGTAGA	Brain or muscle tissues	Pigs	Turčeková et al., 2013
Nested PCR	B1	S1: TGTTCTGTCCTATCGCAACG AS1: ACGGATGCAGTTCCTTTCTG S2: TCTTCCCAGACGTGGATTTC AS2: CTCGACAATACGCTGCTTGA	Blood	Rabbits	Shin et al., 2013
Nested-PCR	B1	Fi: GGAACTGCATCCGTTCATGAG Ri: TCTTTAAAGCGTTCGTGGTC Ro: TGCATAGGTTGCAGTCACTG Ro: GGCGACCAATCTGCGAATACACC	Blood	Dogs and cats	Lee et al., 2008
Conventional PCR	B1	GGAACTGCATCCGTTCATGAG TCTTTAAAGCGTTCGTGGTC	Muscle tissues	Pigs	Hill et al., 2006
Conventional PCR	B1	GGAACTGCATCCGTTCATGAG CTTTAAAGCGTTCGTGGTC	Milk	Sheep	Fusco et al., 2007
Conventional PCR	B1	Tg1: AAAAATGTGGGAATGAAAGAG Tg2: ACGAATCAACGGAACTGTAAT	Blood	Pigs	Ortega et al., 2013
Conventional PCR	B1	B22: AACGGGCGAGTAGCACCTGAGGAGA B23: TGGGTCTACGTCGATGGCATGACAAC	Heart tissue	Sheep	Boughattas et al., 2014

1.2. Specimen Collection

All specimens for DNA extraction should be collected in a highly hygienic way. It is important to preserve the samples at 4°C until DNA extraction and if possible, proceed to the extraction as soon as possible. When a specimen is not correctly preserved, the material to evaluate could be in an inadequate condition for the PCR (decomposition, degradation, etc). Tachyzoites are extremely and rapidly subject to degradation at ambient temperature (Varlet-Marie et al., 2011), even in nutritive media such as *in vitro* cultivation media or biological fluids.

This may occur during the transport to the laboratories or even during manipulations on the bench; this implies that all sample handling should be carried out on ice and any temporary storage of the samples should be preserved at +4°C.

1.3. Nucleic Acid/DNA Extraction Procedures

It is important to consider the sort of the clinical sample to be purified. For tissue or blood samples, an adequate lysis, efficient protein and lipid elimination is imperative together with a good DNA solubilization, to guarantee a good quality material for evaluation. The uses of commercial kits, based mainly in chromatography, are very good options to perform the DNA extraction for these kind of samples. On the other hand, in the case of CFS for example, the method of lysis centrifugation has been reported as a good option (Alfonso et al., 2008).

It is important to consider around 1 mL of the sample in liquid form to process to increase the probability to detect the presence of the parasite (Jalal et al., 2004).

In a multicentric study from France, laboratories with experience on DNA extraction were asked to describe their commercial kits used for *T. gondii*. Qiagen products were by far the most frequently used, although it is not known whether this was based on scientific grounds or a result of the better commercial strategy of this supplier (Sterkers et al., 2010). In general, in France very fewf laboratories preferred the "laboratory-developed" methods, including Tween-Nonidet NaOH method (TNN) and Chelex resin, instead of commercialized kits. It is important to choose the appropriate DNA extraction method, because it may affect PCR assays in different ways (Edvinsson et al., 2004).

1.4. PCR Targets for *T. gondii*

As previously described (table 1), the most commonly used target for PCR detection is the 35-fold repetitive B1 gene (Burg et al., 1989), highly conserved among *Toxoplasma* strains. Another single-copy of sequences used is the SAG-1 (P-30), which has been shown to be a satisfactory PCR target for the detection of *T. gondii.* Likewise, the SAG-2, SAG-3, GRA-4 and ROP-1 genes have been used as PCR targets in research laboratories (Contini et al., 2006).

1.5. *T. gondii* Amplification Protocols with Gel-Based Detection

For *T. gondii* detection by endpoint PCR, several reports have been published, many of them focused for detecting amplicon targets in B1 gene (Burg et al., 1989) or 529 repeat element; they also compared the efficiency of detection from the different types of clinical samples (Bretange et al., 1993; Guy et al., 1996; Cresti et al., 2001; Chabbert et al., 2004; Cermáková et al., 2005; Nowakowska et al., 2002; Gandhoke et a., 2009; Cermáková et al., 2009; Mesquita et al., 2010a; Pinganelli et al., 2012; Lee et al., 2012; Mikita et al., 2013; Sugita et al., 2013; Asai et al., 2013; Delahes et al., 2013).

The End-point PCR as well as the nested PCR protocols are amplification methods that need the visualization with electrophoresis to evidence the final results.

The End-point product measurement can be accomplished through the use of fluorescent intercalating dyes, (i.e., ethidium bromide or SYBRGreen) or through measurement of incorporated radioactivity by autoradiography or phosphor imaging.

Hybridization based protocols, such as Southern blots or fluorescence detection are also used. A third type of End-point product measurement uses solid-state approaches in which a bound enzyme produces fluorescence or luminescence.

Also, some laboratories measure the production of amplification products following resolution by HPLC or capillary electrophoresis (Freeman et al., 1999).

However, these methods require post-PCR manipulation for analysis, and could be time and resource consuming, for that reason have now largely been replaced by RT-PCR methods (Smith and Osborn, 2009).

1.6. Real Time PCR *T. gondii* Amplification Protocols

The Real-time quantitative PCR (qPCR) technique provides a rapid, sensitive and quantitative way to detect of a variety of pathogens including *Toxoplasma gondii* (Costa et al., 2000; Lin et al., 2000). The qPCR include faster testing and reduced the possibly sample contamination because the assay is performed in a closed-tube format (Lalonde and Gajadhar, 2011). The main advantages of real-time PCR are its ability to quantify the infection load of a clinical specimen and its long linear range over at least 6 logs of DNA concentrations. Have been demonstrated that qPCR of the B1 gene is extremely sensitive (0.05 parasite/reaction) and highly reproducible (mean interassay CV of 0.4%) (Lin et al., 2000).

The qPCR technology with SYBR Green or TaqMan methodology have been employed for the molecular detection of toxoplasmas and stage differentiations (Costa et al., 2000; Kupferschmidt et al., 2001; Contini et al., 2005; Kompalic-Cristo et al., 2007; Tonini et al., 2010) in a variety of patients and clinical settings. These based fluorescence assay have the advantages over PCR assays to require less manipulation (Contini et al., 2005) and improves the sensitivity and specificity of the test. However, the disadvantage of SYBR Green chemistry is that it detects all double-stranded DNA, including non-specific reaction products. A well-optimized reaction is therefore essential for accurate results. TaqMan methodology it is most commonly brand used because their fluorogenic probe enables the detection of a specific PCR product as it accumulates during PCR cycles.

Moreover, the use of hybridization probes is a mandatory step to reach final and specific results. TaqMan assays have shown a high sensitivity and reproducibility at 100 fg of *T. gondii* DNA (representing a simple parasite) despite differences in diverse biological samples (Jauregui et al., 2001; Kompalic-Cristo et al., 2007).

At the B.C Lab from CIR Biomedicas/UADY, we have demonstrated that the reproducibility of *Toxoplasma* qPCR TaqMan assays is good (Figure 1) and allow detect very small amounts of DNA parasite load. Detailed methodology is described below. It was estimated the sensitivity of the test, and amplifications of 10-fold serial dilutions of DNA *T. gondii* tachyzoites were performed. Dilutions containing from $1x10^5$ to $1x10^{-2}$ DNA tachyzoites, demonstrated positive signals (Ct values) except in $1x10^{-1}$ and $1x10^{-2}$. The Ct values, ranging from 21.27 +/- 0.03 for $1x10^5$ to 36.77 +/- 1.74 for $1x10^0$, showed reproducible linearity over a wide range of DNA *T. gondii* tachyzoites concentration (R^2= 0.965).

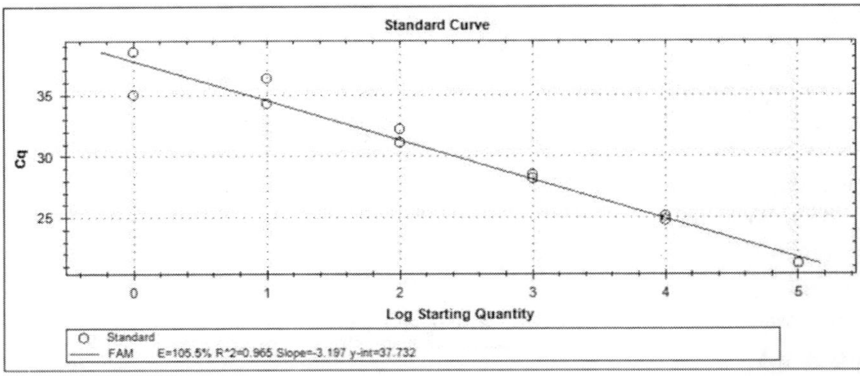

Figure 1. Real-time PCR TaqMan standard curve generated from threshold cycle (Ct) values for DNA *T. gondii* tachyzoites serially diluted from $1x10^5$ to $1x10^{-2}$.

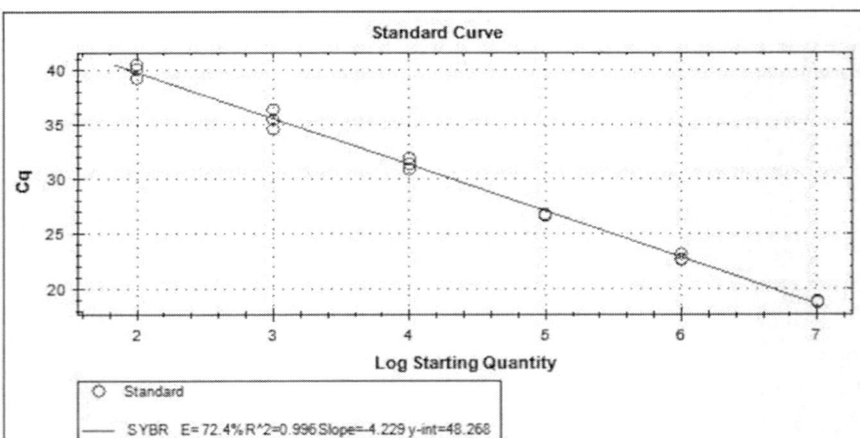

Figure 2. Real-time PCR (qPCR) SYBR Green standard curve generated from threshold cycle (*Ct*) values for DNA *T. gondii* tachyzoites serially diluted from $10x10^6$ to $1x10^{-3}$.

In this chapter it is also described a qPCR using SYBR Green methodology, but should be noted that results are less sensitive compared with the also cited TaqMan assay. Limit detection was $1x10^2$ tachyzoites *vs* $1x10^0$ from SYBR Green and TaqMan assay respectively. However, the standard curve with Ct values, ranging from 18.95 +/- 0.02 for $10x10^6$ to 40.30 +/- 0.23 for $1x10^2$, showed reproducible linearity over a wide range of DNA *T. gondii* tachyzoites concentration (R^2=0.996) (Figure 2).

1.7. Discussion

T. gondii is an important pathogen of significant medical and economical importance to humans and animals, able to cause abortion, congenital disease and several clinical complications in immunosuppressed subjects. The protozoon is globally distributed as an obligate intracellular parasite with a complex lifecycle that favors his maintenance in several species of hosts (definitive and incidentals including humans). The conventional diagnosis tools such as serological evaluations are able to give information about the exposition of the patient and in some successfully cases the parasite can be isolated from *in vivo* or *in vitro* methods. However, the molecular biology tools provide another important gamma of options for a quick and sensitive method to detect the parasite.

All the molecular options (based in PCR technique and its variants) have their own advantages and disadvantages. The conventional PCR is just for detection (presence or absence of DNA in a clinical sample) but is a little time consuming because the electrophoresis after PCR is needed. The nested PCR can detect the presence of *T. gondii* DNA with a greater sensitivity but need to be performed just by experienced operators because the risk of contamination is even high than other PCR variants.

Finally the real time PCR, is a variant of PCR which allows to detect not only the presence of the parasite, but is also able to record the amplification kinetic and estimate of the parasite load in an evaluated sample, with a significant reduction of time for the management of the samples and less probability of carry over contamination. However, the cost of each test is more expensive than conventional or nested PCR and specialized equipment is needed.

For clinical samples, RT-PCR techniques that include an internal probe are the more efficient to detect very small amounts of the parasite. Protocols for RT-PCR using SYBRGreen are efficient for detecting larger quantities of parasites in the samples tested, and can be used a very efficient way for the detection of samples in animals that were inoculated artificially for instance, or in clinical samples where a potentially significant amount of the parasite can be found (ie heart tissue, lymph nodes or brain). This type of technique is not advisable for the detection of parasite in blood samples, amniotic fluid or CFS. The demonstration of low parasite loads in a large proportion of infected AF samples (<10 tachyzoites per mL) (Costa et al., 2001; Romand et al., 2004) makes it necessary to test sensitivity with low Toxoplasma concentration.

To acquire efficient parasite detection, it is recommended to follow quality control practices in the laboratory. When a sample is going to be evaluated for molecular detection of *T. gondii,* it is crucial to preserve the clinical sample at low temperatures (at least at 4ºC) (Varlet-Marie et al., 2011) because the parasite DNA it is prone to rapid degradation.

Also it is important to choose an efficient method of DNA purification that allows to recover a good amount of material for evaluation in an easy and affordable format, free of contaminants or residuals which can act as inhibitors during the DNA *T. gondii* detection.

It is important to consider the species when clinical samples are evaluated; for example in the case of purifying blood samples of pork with commercial kits in column format, it may involve major episodes of centrifugation as the proportion of the blood components is not the same as in other species. Centrifuging of the sample is required as often as necessary until the samples pass through the membrane of the column; this methodology can be successfully used for *T.gondii*. In the case of meat, there are methodologies that include magnetic capture of parasite DNA, which significantly increase the efficiency of detection in the samples tested; so for meat samples, this methodology is a very attractive option that allows detection more accuracy, as demonstrated in different domestic species (Opsteegh et al., 2010; Opsteegh et al., 2011; Juránková et al., 2013; Juránková et al., 2014a; Juránková et al., 2014b).

It is highly recommended to always be included appropiated DNA *–T gondii* amplification controls (in every round of amplification), preferably obtained from reference strains. Always the viability of DNA samples being analyzed; either with internal amplification control or by a housekeeper gene amplification should be evaluated.

Also, all procedures for the detection of *T. gondii* DNA *should be* performed in separate areas, preferably in a pre-PCR (room 1) area where only the "mastermix" (white area) will be prepared, a second area (room 2) where should perform both: the purification of DNA, such as the addition of purified samples of DNA to the master-mix prepared in the room 1, and a third area (room 3), which must be the equipment to perform and analyze the methodologies needed (cyclers, electrophoresis chambers, UV photo documentation system, UV transilluminator, etc.), to avoid carry over contamination and thus avoid false positive results.

Detection of DNA of *T. gondii* may not be easy, but the use of all the tools of molecular biology available, which allow detection of the parasite, can be implemented in any laboratory with equipment and trained personnel following the standards of quality control protocols. The molecular techniques will be able, without difficulty to detect the presence and parasite load in different kind of samples in both humans and animals, providing more information to the epidemiologists, infectious disease specialists and other professionals from the health area.

2. MATERIALS

2.1. Isolation of DNA from blood and tissue samples	Buffers (DNeasy Blood and Tissue Kit, QIAGEN) Lysis buffer AL: Contains mainly 10 mM Tris-HCL, pH 7.5, 5mM $MgCl_2$, 0.32 mM saccharosa and Tritin X-100 1% v/v) Buffer ATL* Buffer AW1 Buffer AW2 Buffer AE Proteinase K Ethanol (96–100%) PBS, pH 7.2 (50 mM potassium phosphate, 150 mM NaCl) Consumables Pipets and pipet tips Vortexer Microcentrifuge tubes (1.5 ml or 2 ml) Microcentrifuge with rotor for 1.5 ml and 2 ml tubes Thermomixer, shaking water bath, or rocking platform for heating at 56°C *Buffer only for tissue samples

3. METHODS

3.1. Isolation of DNA from biological samples	Modified by Jalal et al. (2004) Make aliquot of blood (1mL) into 2-mL microcentrifuge tubes Dispense 500mL lysis buffer AL Vortex Incubate on ice for 5 min
Blood samples	Centrifuge at 8000 g for 3 min Remove supernatant Pellet resuspend in 0.1mL lysis buffer Centrifuge at 8000 g for 3 min Supernatants from the 2 tubes are combined to give a total volume of 0.2 mL
	Follow the protocol of DNeasy Blood and Tissue Kit, (QIAGEN) Pipet 20 µl proteinase K into a 1.5 ml or 2 ml micro centrifuge tube. Add 200 µl of supernatants above Mix thoroughly by vortexing, and incubate at 56°C for 10 min Add 200 µl ethanol (96–100%) to the sample, and mix thoroughly by vortexing Pipet the mixture into the DNeasy Mini spin column placed in a 2 ml collection tube. Centrifuge at 6000 g (8000 rpm) for 1 min Discard flow-through and collection tube Place the DNeasy Mini spin column in a new 2 ml collection tube, add 500 µl Buffer AW1, and centrifuge for 1 min at 6000 g (8000 rpm) Discard flow-through and collection tuve Place the DNeasy Mini spin column in a new 2 ml collection tube, add 500 µl Buffer AW2, and centrifuge for 3 min at 20,000 g (14,000 rpm) to dry the DNeasy membrane. Discard flow-through and collection tube. Place the DNeasy Mini spin column in a clean 1.5 ml or 2 ml microcentrifuge tube, and pipet 100 µl Buffer AE directly onto the DNeasy membrane. Incubate at room temperature for 1 min, and then centrifuge for 1 min at 6000 g (8000 rpm) to elute.
Tissue samples	According to the *protocol* described by Dubey (1998) Tissue samples (50g) are homogenized in five volumes (w/v) of sterile saline solution, in a blender for 30s at top speed. Add 250 mL of warm (37°C) pepsin-HCl solution (2.6 g of pepsin; 5.0 g of NaC1; 7.0 mL of HCl and distilled water to make 500 mL, pH 1.10- 1.20) Incubate in a shaking water bath for 1 h at 37°C Filter the homogenate through two layers of gauze and centrifuge at 1200 g for 10min Remove supernatant

	Pellet resuspend in 20mL of PBS (pH 7.2) Neutralize the homogenate with 15mL of 1.2% sodium bicarbonate (pH 8.3) After mixing, centrifuge at 1200 g for 10min From the resulting pellet, one aliquot (25mg) is digested overnight at 55°C with 180 µl digestion buffer ATL. (The rest of the pellet can be used for inoculation in mice). Follow the protocol of DNeasy Blood and Tissue Kit, (QIAGEN) Add 20 µl proteinase K. Mix thoroughly by vortexing, and incubate at 56°C until the tissue is completely lysed. Vortex occasionally during incubation to disperse the sample, or place in a thermomixer, shaking water bath, or on a rocking platform. Vortex for 15 s. Add 200 µl Buffer AL to the sample, and mix thoroughly by vortexing. Then add 200 µl ethanol (96–100%), and mix again thoroughly by vortexing. Pipet the mixture from step 3 (including any precipitate) into the DNeasy Mini spin column placed in a 2 ml collection tube (provided). Centrifuge at _6000 x g (8000 rpm) for 1 min. Discard flow-through and collection tube. Place the DNeasy Mini spin column in a new 2 ml collection tube (provided), add 500 µl Buffer AW1, and centrifuge for 1 min at _6000 x g (8000 rpm). Discard flow-through and collection tube. Place the DNeasy Mini spin column in a new 2 ml collection tube (provided), add 500 µl Buffer AW2, and centrifuge for 3 min at 20,000 x g (14,000 rpm) to dry the DNeasy membrane. Discard flow-through and collection tube. Place the DNeasy Mini spin column in a clean 1.5 ml or 2 ml microcentrifuge tube (not provided), and pipet 200 µl Buffer AE directly onto the DNeasy membrane. Incubate at room temperature for 1 min, and then centrifuge for 1 min at 6000 x g (8000 rpm) to elute.

3.1. Protocol for End Point PCR, Target B1 Gene

The PCR procedures (described the first by Mezquita *et al,* 2010b and the second by Jalal et al., 2004) is performed in three rooms. This is done to minimize the danger of contamination of buffers, primers, patient samples, etc. with PCR products (amplimers).

Work in *room 1*

1. Thaw all PCR solutions at room temperature or on ice (keep enzymes at 4 °C). Short vortex and spin before use.
2. Prepare the number of mixes needed according to mix for End Point PCR.
3. Aliquot the mix to vials with each 20 uL per vial.
4. Short spin, 15 s 11,000 × *g* .
5. Store in small plastic bags (seal) and take them to *room 2* for direct use or store in clean −20 °C freezer for later use (can be stored for 3 months).

Primers (B22-B23) from B1 gene (expected amplicon size of 115 bp)

Forward	B22	AACGGGCGAGTAGCACCTGAGGAGA
Reverse	B23	TGGGTCTACGTCGATGGCATGACAAC

Conditions for B22 and B23 primers

Solutions Conventional PCR	End concentration
dNTP	200uM of each dNTP
$MgCl_2$	1.0 mM
Forward	20uM
Reverse	20uM
RNase-free H_2O	the required amount to complete the reaction volume
Taq polymerase	1U of GoTaq enzime Hot Star Polymerase
Mix volume	20uL
DNA sample	5uL
Total volume	25uL

Work in *room 3* with thermocycler

1. Thaw all PCR mixes at room temperature. Short vortex and spin before use.
2. Number the vials.
3. Add 5 uL isolated nucleic acid per patient sample. For negative control add 5 uL of RNase-free H_2O. For positive control add 5 uL of known positive patient DNA.
4. Close all vials well and place in the PCR machine after a short spin.

The PCR cycling program for B22 and B23 primers is as follows:

Program	Cycles	Temperature (°C)	Time
Initial denaturation		95	5 min
Denaturation	35	95	1 min
Annealing		61	1 min
Extension		72	1 min
Final extension		72	5 min

Primers (Tg1-Tg2) from B1 gene (expected amplicon size of 469 bp)

Forward	Tg1	AAAAATGTGGGAATGAAAGAG
Reverse	Tg2	ACGAATCAACGGAACTGTAAT

Conditions for Tg1 and Tg2 primers

Solutions Conventional PCR	End concentration
dNTP	200uL of each dNTP
$MgCl_2$	0.8uM
Forward	20uM
Rereverse	20uM
RNase-free H_2O	the required amount to complete the reaction volume
Taq polymerase	1U of GoTaq enzyme Hot Star Polymerase
Mix volume	22uL
DNA sample	3uL
Total volume	25uL

The PCR cycling program for Tg1 and Tg2 primers is as follows:

After thermal cycles, PCR products were electrophoresed in 2% agarose gel and stained with ethidium bromide. DNA fragments were visualized under UV illumination.

3.2. Real Time qPCR on B1 Gene of *T. Gondii*

Taqman Methodology

Primers and TaqMan probe for the B1 gene of *T. gondii* have been previously described by Kompalic-Cristo et al., (2007). (expected amplicon size of 62 bp).

Work in *room 1*

1. Thaw all PCR solutions at room temperature or on ice (keep enzymes at 4 °C). Short vortex and spin before use.
2. Prepare the number of mixes needed according to mix for real-time *T. gondii* PCR.
3. Transfer 21 uL of PCR reaction mix into well a 96 –well reaction plate.
4. Store in small plastic bags (seal) and take them to *room 2* for direct use or store in clean −20 °C freezer for later use (can be stored for 3 months).

Program	Cycles	Temperature (°C)	Time
Initial denaturation		94	5 min
Denaturation	35	94	45 sec
annealing		50	30 sec
Extension		72	1 min
Final extension		72	7 min

Forward	5′CTAGTATCGTGCGGCAATGTG 3′
Reverse	5′GGCAGCGTCTCTTCCTCTTTT 3′
Probe	5′(6-FAM)-CCACCTCGCCTCTTGG-(NFQ-MGB) 3′

Work in *room 3* with thermocycler

1. Add 4 uL isolated nucleic acid per patient sample. For negative control add 4 uL of RNase-free H_2O. For positive control add 4 uL of known positive patient DNA.
2. Seal the plate with the appropriate cover.
3. Centrifuge the plate briefly.
4. Load the plate into the instrument.

The real-time PCR cycling program is as follows:

PCR mixture ingredients *T. gondii* real-time PCR	uL per sample (1x)
RNase-free H_2O	5.01
1x TaqMan Universal PCR Master mix (PE Applied Biosystems)	12.5
$MgCl_2$ is included in Mastermix -- 5mM end concentration	
Primers Forward (0.90uM)	1.12
Primers Reverse (0.90uM)	1.12
Flourscein-labeled probe (0.25 uM)	1.25
DNA isolate sample	4uL
Total volume	25

<table>
<tr><th>Program</th><th>Cycles</th><th>Temperature (°C)</th><th>Time</th></tr>
<tr><td>UNG incubation</td><td rowspan="4">40</td><td>50</td><td>2 min</td></tr>
<tr><td>Polymerase activation</td><td>95</td><td>10 min</td></tr>
<tr><td>Denature</td><td>95</td><td>15 s</td></tr>
<tr><td>Annel/Extend</td><td>60</td><td>1 min</td></tr>
</table>

The program takes about 2 h and 3 min.

SYBER Green Methodology

Primers used (described Burg et al., 1989) for this RT PCR an amplification of a region for B1 gene is performed (Implemented in RT by Hernandez-Cortazar., 2013).

Work in *room 1*

1. Thaw all PCR solutions at room temperature or on ice (keep enzymes at 4 °C). Short vortex and spin before use.
2. Prepare the number of mixes needed according to mix for real-time *T. gondii* PCR.
3. Transfer 15 uL of PCR reaction mix into well a 96 –well reaction plate.
4. Store in small plastic bags (seal) and take them to *room 2* for direct use or store in clean −20 °C freezer for later use (can be stored for 3 months).

Forward B22	AACGGGCGAGTAGCACCTGAGGAGA
Reverse B23	TGGGTCTACGTCGATGGCATGACAAC

PCR mixture *T. gondii* real-time PCR	uL per sample (1x)
SsoAdvanced^{TM} SYBR Green Supermix (Bio-Rad)	10
RNase-free H_2O	3
Primers Forward	1
Primers Reverse	1
DNA isolate sample	5uL
Total volume	20

Work in *room 3* with thermocycler

1. Add 5 uL isolated nucleic acid per patient sample. For negative control add 5 uL of RNase-free H_2O. For positive control add 5 uL of known positive patient DNA.
2. Seal the plate with the appropriate cover.
3. Centrifuge the plate briefly.
4. Load the plate into the instrument.

The real-time PCR cycling program is as follows:

3.2.1. Interpretation of Results (as Performed on a CFX96™ Real-Time PCR)

For the absolute quantitative interpretation of the CFX96™ Real-Time PCR (BioRad), results are assisted by the sequence detector software (CFX Manager™ software) by interpolation from the standard curve expressed as the threshold cycle value (Ct), i.e., the number of cycle at which a significant fluorescence signal is observed in a given positive sample.

Program	Cycles	Temperature (°C)	Time
Initial denaturation		95	3 min
Denaturation	40	95	10 s
Annel/Extend		60	30 s

REFERENCES

Alfonso Y., Fraga J., Cox R., Bandera F., Pomier O., Fonseca C., Ginorio D., Torres G., Capo V. Comparison of four DNA extraction methods from cerebrospinal fluid for the detection of Toxoplasma gondii by polymerase chain reaction in AIDS patients. *Med. Sci. Monit.,* 2008 Mar.;14(3): MT1-6.

Alfonso Y., Fraga J., Cox R., Jiménez N., Capó V., Pomier O., Fonseca C., Bandera F., Dorta-Contreras A. J., Calá V., Ginorio D. Conventional polymerase chain reaction for the diagnosis of neurotoxoplasmosis: comparison of three sets of primers for the B1 gene using CSF samples. *Diagn. Microbiol. Infect. Dis.*, 2013.75:150-4.

Al-Qassab S., Reichel M. P., Su C., Jenkins D., Hall C., Windsor P. A., Dubey J. P., Ellis J. Isolation of Toxoplasma gondii from the brain of a dog in Australia and its biological and molecular characterization. *Vet. Parasitol.,* 2009 Oct. 14;164(2-4):335-9.

Asai T. [The diagnosis of toxoplasmic encephalitis by polymerase chain reaction]. *Rinsho Shinkeigaku.*, 2013;53(11):1194-5.

Asgari Q., Fekri M., Monabati A., Kalantary M., Mohammadpour I., Motazedian M. H., Sarkari B. Molecular Genotyping of Toxoplasma gondii in Human Spontaneous Aborted Fetuses in Shiraz, Southern Iran. *Iran. J. Public Health*, 2013 Jun. 1;42(6):620-5. eCollection 2013.

Baquero-Artigao F., del Castillo Martín F., Fuentes Corripio I., Goncé Mellgren A., Fortuny Guasch C., de la Calle Fernández-Miranda M., González-Tomé M. I., Couceiro Gianzo J. A., Neth O., Ramos Amador J. T.; Grupo de Trabajo de Infección Congénita y Perinatal de la Sociedad Española de Infectología Pediátrica (SEIP). [The Spanish Society of Pediatric Infectious Diseases Guidelines for the diagnosis and treatment of congenital toxoplasmosis]. *An. Pediatr. (Barc).,* 2013 Aug.;79(2):116.e1-116.e16.

Berger-Schoch A. E., Herrmann D. C., Schares G., Müller N., Bernet D., Gottstein B., Frey C. F. Prevalence and genotypes of Toxoplasma gondii in feline faeces (oocysts) and meat from sheep, cattle and pigs in Switzerland. *Vet. Parasitol.*, 2011 May 11;177(3-4):290-7.

Boughattas S., Ayari K., Sa T., Aoun K., Bouratbine A. Survey of the Parasite Toxoplasma gondii in Human Consumed Ovine Meat in Tunis City. *PLoS One,* 2014. 9.

Bretagne S., Costa J. M., Vidaud M., Tran J., Nhieu V., Fleury-Feith J. Detection of Toxoplasma gondii by competitive DNA amplification of bronchoalveolar lavage samples. *J. Infect. Dis.*, 1993 Dec.;168(6):1585-8.

Buchbinder S., Blatz R., Rodloff A. C. (2003): Comparison of real-time PCR detection methods for B1 and P30 genes of Toxoplasma gondii. *Diagn. Microbiol. Infect. Dis.*, 45, 4: 269-271.

Burg J. L., Grover C. M., Pouletty P., Boothroyd J. C. Direct and sensitive detection of a pathogenic protozoan, Toxoplasma gondii, by polymerase chain reaction. *J. Clin. Microbiol.*, 1989 Aug.;27(8):1787-92.

Caner A., Döşkaya M., Karasu Z., Değirmenci A., Guy E., Kiliç M., Zeytunlu M., Francis J., Bozoklar A., Gürüz Y. Incidence and diagnosis of active toxoplasma infection among liver transplant recipients in Western Turkey. *Liver Transpl.*, 2008 Oct.;14(10):1526-32.

Cardona N., de-la-Torre A., Siachoque H., Patarroyo M. A., Gomez-Marin J. E. (2009): Toxoplasma gondii: P30 peptides recognition pattern in human toxoplasmosis. *Exp. Parasitol.*, 123, 2: 199-202.

Cermáková Z., Prásil P., Valenta Z., Förstl M., Plísková L., Bolehovská R. [Considering the role of the PCR method in routine diagnosis of toxoplasmosis in peripheral blood tests in immunocompetent patients]. *Klin. Mikrobiol. Infekc. Lek.*, 2009 Aug.;15(4):138-42.

Cermáková Z., Rysková O., Plísková L. Polymerase chain reaction for detection of Toxoplasma gondii in human biological samples. *Folia Microbiol., (Praha).* 2005;50(4):341-4.

Chabbert E., Lachaud L., Crobu L., Bastien P. Comparison of two widely used PCR primer systems for detection of toxoplasma in amniotic fluid, blood, and tissues. *J. Clin. Microbiol.*, 2004 Apr.;42(4):1719-22.

Chabbert E., Lachaud L., Crobu L., Bastien P. Comparison of two widely used PCR primer systems for detection of toxoplasma in amniotic fluid, blood, and tissues. *J. Clin. Microbiol.,* 2004 Apr.;42(4):1719-22.

Correia C. C., Melo H. R., Costa V. M. (2010): Influence of neurotoxoplasmosis characteristics on real-time PCR sensitivity among AIDS patients in Brazil. *Trans. R. Soc. Trop. Med. Hyg.,* 104, 1: 24-28.

Costa, J. M., Ernault, P., Gautier, E. and Bretagne, S. (2001) Prenatal diagnosis of congenital toxoplasmosis by duplex real-time PCR using fluorescence resonance energy transfer hybridization probes. *Prenat. Diagn.,* 21, 85-88.

Cresti S., Ciacci C., Donati E., Giordano I., Tordini G., Barberi A. Evaluation of PCR methods for 5S-rDNA and p30 genes to detect Toxoplasma gondii in blood and other clinical samples. *New Microbiol.,* 2001 Apr.;24(2): 171-4.

da Silva R. C., Langoni H., Su C., da Silva A. V. (2011): Genotypic characterization of Toxoplasma gondii in sheep from Brazilian slaughterhouses: new atypical genotypes and the clonal type II strain identified. *Vet. Parasitol.*, 175, 1-2: 173-177.

Dehkordi F. S., Borujeni M. R., Rahimi E., Abdizadeh R. Detection of Toxoplasma gondii in raw caprine, ovine, buffalo, bovine, and camel milk using cell cultivation, cat bioassay, capture ELISA, and PCR methods in Iran. *Foodborne Pathog. Dis.*, 2013 Feb.;10(2):120-5.

Delhaes L., Yera H., Ache S., Tsatsaris V., Houfflin-Debarge V. Contribution of molecular diagnosis to congenital toxoplasmosis. *Diagn. Microbiol. Infect. Dis.,* 2013 Jun.;76(2):244-7.

Dubey J. P., Moura L., Majumdar D., Sundar N., Velmurugan G. V., Kwok O. C., Kelly P., Krecek R. C., Su C. Isolation and characterization of viable Toxoplasma gondii isolates revealed possible high frequency of mixed infection in feral cats (Felis domesticus) from St Kitts, West Indies. *Parasitology*, 2009 May;136(6):589-94.

Dubey J. P. Duration of immunity to shedding of Toxoplasma gondii oocysts by cats. *J. Parasitol.*, 1995 Jun.;81(3):410-5.

Dubey J. P. Toxoplasma Gondii. In: Baron S, editor. Medical Microbiology. 4th edition. Galveston (TX): University of Texas Medical Branch at Galveston; 1996. Chapter 84.

Edvinsson B., Jalal S., Nord C. E., Pedersen B. S., Evengård B.; ECSMID Study Group on Toxoplasmosis. DNA extraction and PCR assays for detection of Toxoplasma gondii. *APMIS,* 2004 Jun.;112(6):342-8.

Edvinsson, Benjamin. Molecular diagnosis of infection with Toxoplasma gondii in immunocompromised patients. Thesis. Karolinska Institute. 2006. Available at http://hdl.handle.net/10616/39302

Eida O. M., Eida M. M., Ahmed A. B. (2009): Evaluation of polymerase chain reaction on amniotic fluid for diagnosis of congenital toxoplasmosis. *J. Egypt Soc. Parasitol.,* 39, 2: 541-550.

Fallahi Sh., Kazemi B., Seyyed tabaei S. J., Bandehpour M., Lasjerdi Z., Taghipour N., Zebardast N., Nikmanesh B., Omrani V. F., Ebrahimzadeh F. Comparison of the RE and B1 gene for detection of Toxoplasma gondii infection in children with cancer. *Parasitol. Int.,* 2014 Feb;63(1):37-41.

Freeman W. M., Walker S. J., Vrana K. E. Quantitative RT-PCR: pitfalls and potential. *Biotechniques,* 1999 Jan.;26(1):112-22, 124-5.

Fusco G., Rinaldi L., Guarino A., Proroga Y. T., Pesce A., Giuseppina de M., Cringoli G. Toxoplasma gondii in sheep from the Campania region (Italy). *Vet. Parasitol.*, 2007 Nov. 10;149(3-4):271-4.

Gandhoke I., Aggarwal R., Hussain S. A., Pasha S. T., Sethi P., Thakur S., Lal S., Khare S. Congenital CMV infection; diagnosis in symptomatic infants. *Indian J. Med. Microbiol.*, 2009 Jul.-Sep.;27(3):222-5.

Guy E. C., Pelloux H., Lappalainen M., Aspöck H., Hassl A., Melby K. K., Holberg-Pettersen M., Petersen E., Simon J., Ambroise-Thomas P. Interlaboratory comparison of polymerase chain reaction for the detection of Toxoplasma gondii DNA added to samples of amniotic fluid. *Eur. J. Clin. Microbiol. Infect. Dis.*, 1996 Oct.;15(10):836-9.

Hierl T., Reischl U., Lang P., Hebart H., Stark M., Kyme P., Autenrieth I. B. Preliminary evaluation of one conventional nested and two real-time PCR assays for the detection of Toxoplasma gondii in immunocompromised patients. *J. Med. Microbiol.*, 2004 Jul.;53(Pt 7):629-32.

Hill D. E., Chirukandoth S., Dubey J. P., Lunney J. K., Gamble H. R. Comparison of detection methods for Toxoplasma gondii in naturally and experimentally infected swine. *Vet. Parasitol.*, 2006 Oct. 10;141(1-2): 9-17.

Ivović V., Vujanic M., Zivkovic T., Klun I., Djurkovic-Djaković O. Molecular detection and genotyping of T. gondii from clinical samples. Chapter 5. Toxoplasmosis. Recent Advances. Intech. Pp. 103-120.

Jalal S., Nord C. E., Lappalainen M., Evengård B.; ESCMID Study Group on Toxoplasmosis.Rapid and sensitive diagnosis of Toxoplasma gondii infections by PCR. *Clin. Microbiol. Infect.*, 2004 Oct.;10 (10):937-9.

Jones C. D., Okhravi N., Adamson P., Tasker S., Lightman S. Comparison of PCR detection methods for B1, P30, and 18S rDNA genes of T. gondii in aqueous humor. *Invest. Ophthalmol. Vis. Sci.*, 2000 Mar.;41(3):634-44.

Juránková J., Basso W., Neumayerová H., Baláž V., Jánová E., Sidler X., Deplazes P., Koudela B. Brain is the predilection site of Toxoplasma gondii in experimentally inoculated pigs as revealed by magnetic capture and real-time PCR. *Food Microbiol.*, 2014a Apr.;38:167-70.

Juránková J., Hůrková-Hofmannová L., Volf J., Baláž V., Piálek J. Efficacy of magnetic capture in comparison with conventional DNA isolation in a survey of Toxoplasma gondii in wild house mice. *Eur. J. Protistol.*, 2014b Feb.;50(1):11-5.

Juránková J., Opsteegh M., Neumayerová H., Kovařčík K., Frencová A., Baláž V., Volf J., Koudela B. Quantification of Toxoplasma gondii in tissue samples of experimentally infected goats by magnetic capture and real-time PCR. *Vet. Parasitol.*, 2013 Mar. 31;193(1-3):95-9.

Kompalic-Cristo A., Frotta C., Suárez-Mutis M., Fernandes O., Britto C. Evaluation of a real-time PCR assay based on the repetitive B1 gene for the detection of Toxoplasma gondii in human peripheral blood. *Parasitol. Res.*, 2007 Aug.;101(3):619-25.

Kravetz J. D., Federman D. G. Toxoplasmosis in pregnancy. *Am. J. Med.*, 2005 Mar.;118(3):212-6.

Lalonde L. F., Gajadhar A. A. Detection and differentiation of coccidian oocysts by real-time PCR and melting curve analysis. *J. Parasitol.*, 2011 Aug.;97(4):725-30.

Lau Y. L., Meganathan P., Sonaimuthu P., Thiruvengadam G., Nissapatorn V., Chen Y. Specific, sensitive, and rapid diagnosis of active toxoplasmosis by a loop-mediated isothermal amplification method using blood samples from patients. *J. Clin. Microbiol.*, 2010 Oct.;48(10):3698-702.

Lee J. Y., Lee S. E., Lee E. G., Song K. H. Nested PCR-based detection of Toxoplasma gondii in German shepherd dogs and stray cats in South Korea. *Res. Vet. Sci.*, 2008 Aug.; 85(1):125-7.

Lee S. E., Hong S. H., Lee S. H., Jeong Y. I., Lim S. J., Kwon O. W., Kim S. H., You Y. S., Cho S. H., Lee W. J. Detection of ocular Toxoplasma gondii infection in chronic irregular recurrent uveitis by PCR. *Korean J. Parasitol.*, 2012 Sep.;50(3):229-31.

Lin M. H., Chen T. C., Kuo T. T., Tseng C. C., Tseng C. P. Real-time PCR for quantitative detection of Toxoplasma gondii. *J. Clin. Microbiol.*, 2000. 38:4121-5.

Lopes-Mori F. M., Mitsuka-Breganó R., Bittencourt L. H., Dias R. C., Gonçalves D. D., Capobiango J. D., Reiche E. M., Morimoto H. K., Freire R. L., Navarro I. T. Gestational toxoplasmosis in Paraná State, Brazil: prevalence of IgG antibodies and associated risk factors. *Braz. J. Infect. Dis.*, 2013 Jul.-Aug.;17(4):405-9.

Mancianti F., Nardoni S., Ariti G., Parlanti D., Giuliani G., Papini R. A. Cross-sectional survey of Toxoplasma gondii infection in colony cats from urban Florence (Italy). *J. Feline Med. Surg.*, 2010 Apr.;12(4):351-4.

Martinez C. E., Zhang D., Conway M. D., Peyman G. A. Successful management of ocular toxoplasmosis during pregnancy using combined intraocular clindamycin and dexamethasone with systemic sulfadiazine. *Int. Ophthalmol.*, 1998-1999;22(2):85-8.

Martino, R., S. Bretagne, et al. (2005). "Early detection of Toxoplasma infection by molecular monitoring of Toxoplasma gondii in peripheral blood samples after allogeneic stem cell transplantation." *Clin. Infect. Dis.*, 40(1): 67-78.

Mesquita R. T., Vidal J. E., Pereira-Chioccola V. L. Molecular diagnosis of cerebral toxoplasmosis: comparing markers that determine Toxoplasma gondii by PCR in peripheral blood from HIV-infected patients. *Braz. J. Infect. Dis.*, 2010a Jul.-Aug.;14(4):346-50.

Mesquita R. T., Ziegler A. P., Hiramoto R. M., Vidal J. E., Pereira-Chioccola V. L. Real-time quantitative PCR in cerebral toxoplasmosis diagnosis of Brazilian human immunodeficiency virus-infected patients. *J. Med. Microbiol.,* 2010b Jun.;59(Pt 6):641-7.

Mikita K., Maeda T., Ono T., Miyahira Y., Asai T., Kawana A. The utility of cerebrospinal fluid for the molecular diagnosis of toxoplasmic encephalitis. *Diagn. Microbiol. Infect. Dis.,* 2013 Feb.;75(2):155-9.

Miller M. A., Grigg M. E., Kreuder C., James E. R., Melli A. C., Crosbie P. R., Jessup D. A., Boothroyd J. C., Brownstein D., Conrad P. A. (2004): An unusual genotype of Toxoplasma gondii is common in California sea otters (Enhydra lutris nereis) and is a cause of mortality. *Int. J. Parasitol.,* 34, 3: 275-284.

Nowakowska D., Gołab E., Czichos E., Krekora M., Wilczyński J. [Detection of Toxoplasma gondii in human placenta by PCR and placental histologic findings]. *Wiad. Parazytol.*, 2002;48(3):301-9.

Okay T. S., Yamamoto L., Oliveira L. C., Manuli E. R., Andrade Junior H. F., Del Negro G. M. (2009):Significant performance variation among PCR systems in diagnosing congenital toxoplasmosis in São Paulo, Brazil: analysis of 467 amniotic fluid samples. *Clinics,* (Sao Paulo) 64, 3: 171-6.

Opsteegh M., Langelaar M., Sprong H., den Hartog L., De Craeye S., Bokken G., Ajzenberg D., Kijlstra A., van der Giessen J. Direct detection and genotyping of Toxoplasma gondii in meat samples using magnetic capture and PCR. *Int. J. Food Microbiol.*, 2010 May 15;139(3):193-201.

Opsteegh M., Teunis P., Züchner L., Koets A., Langelaar M., van der Giessen J. Low predictive value of seroprevalence of Toxoplasma gondii in cattle for detection of parasite DNA. *Int. J. Parasitol.*, 2011 Mar.;41(3-4): 343-54.

Ortega-Pacheco A., Acosta Viana K. Y., Guzmán-Marín E., Segura-Correa J. C., Alvarez-Fleites M., Jiménez-Coello M. Prevalence and risk factors of Toxoplasma gondii in fattening pigs farm from Yucatan, Mexico. *Biomed. Res. Int.,* 2013;2013:231497.

Pardini L., Carral L. A., Bernstein M., Gos M. L., Olejnik P., Unzaga J. M., Kaufer F. J., Freuler C. B., Durlach R. A., Venturini M. C. First isolation and molecular characterization of Toxoplasma gondii from a human placenta in Argentina. *Parasitol. Int.,* 2013 Oct. 25. pii: S1383-5769(13)00171-2.

Pignanelli S. Laboratory diagnosis of Toxoplasma gondii infection with direct and indirect diagnostic techniques. *Indian J. Pathol. Microbiol.*, 2011 Oct.-Dec.;54(4):786-9.

Romand, S., Chosson, M., Franck, J., Wallon, M., Kieffer, F., Kaiser, K., Dumon, H., Peyron, F., Thulliez, P. and Picot, S. (2004) Usefulness of quantitative polymerase chain reaction in amniotic fluid as early prognostic marker of fetal infection with Toxoplasma gondii. *Am. J. Obstet. Gynecol.*, 190, 797-802.

Saadatnia G., Golkar M. A review on human toxoplasmosis. *Scand. J. Infect. Dis.,* 2012 Nov.;44(11):805-14.

Salant H., Spira D. T., Hamburger J. A comparative analysis of coprologic diagnostic methods for detection of *Toxoplama gondii* in cats. *Am. J. Trop. Med. Hyg.*, 2010 May;82(5):865-70.

Shin H. G., Lee S. E., Hong S. H., Kim S. M., Choi Y. K., Park H. J., Seo K. W., Song K. H. Prevalence of Toxoplasma gondii Infection in Rabbits of Korea by Serological Tests and Nested Polymerase Chain Reaction. *J. Vet. Med. Sci.*, 2013 Dec 30;75(12):1609-13.

Smith C. J., Osborn A. M. Advantages and limitations of quantitative PCR (Q-PCR)-based approaches in microbial ecology. *FEMS Microbiol. Ecol.,* 2009 Jan.;67(1):6-20.

Sterkers Y., Varlet-Marie E., Marty P., Bastien P.; ANOFEL Toxoplasma-PCR Quality Control Group. Diversity and evolution of methods and practices for the molecular diagnosis of congenital toxoplasmosis in France: a 4-year survey. *Clin. Microbiol. Infect.*, 2010 Oct;16(10):1594-602.

Sugita S., Ogawa M., Inoue S., Shimizu N., Mochizuki M. Diagnosis of ocular toxoplasmosis by two polymerase chain reaction (PCR) examinations: qualitative multiplex and quantitative real-time. *Jpn. J. Ophthalmol.*, 2011 Sep.;55(5):495-501.

Sugita S., Ogawa M., Shimizu N., Morio T., Ohguro N., Nakai K., Maruyama K., Nagata K., Takeda A., Usui Y., Sonoda K. H., Takeuchi M., Mochizuki M. Use of a comprehensive polymerase chain reaction system for diagnosis of ocular infectious diseases. *Ophthalmology,* 2013 Sep.;120(9):1761-8.

Teixeira L. E., Kanunfre K. A., Shimokawa P. T., Targa L. S., Rodrigues J. C., Domingues W., Yamamoto L., Okay T. S. The performance of four molecular methods for the laboratory diagnosis of congenital toxoplasmosis in amniotic fluid samples. *Rev. Soc. Bras. Med. Trop.,* 2013 Sep.-Oct.;46(5):584-8.

Tenter A. M., Heckeroth A. R., Weiss L. M. Toxoplasma gondii: from animals to humans. Int J Parasitol. 2000 Nov;30(12-13):1217-58. Review. Erratum in: *Int. J. Parasitol.*, 2001 Feb.;31(2):217-20.

Truppel J. H., Reifur L., Montiani-Ferreira F., Lange R. R., de Castro Vilani R. G., Gennari S. M., Thomaz-Soccol, V. (2010): Toxoplasma gondii in Capybara (Hydrochaeris hydrochaeris) antibodies and DNA detected by IFAT and PCR. *Parasitol. Res.,* 107, 1: 141-146.

Turčeková Ľ., Antolová D., Reiterová K., Spišák F. Occurrence and genetic characterization of Toxoplasma gondii in naturally infected pigs. *Acta Parasitol.*, 2013 Sep.;58(3):361-6.

Villard O., Breit L., Cimon B., Franck J., Fricker-Hidalgo H., Godineau N., Houze S., Paris L., Pelloux H., Villena I., Candolfi E.; French National Reference Center for Toxoplasmosis Network. Comparison of four commercially available avidity tests for Toxoplasma gondii-specific IgG antibodies. *Clin. Vaccine Immunol.*, 2013 Feb.;20(2):197-204.

Vujanić M., Ivović V., Kataranovski M., Nikolić A., Bobić B., Klun I., Villena I., Kataranovski D., Djurković Djaković O. (2011): Toxoplasmosis in naturally infected rodents in Belgrade, Serbia. *Vector Borne Zoonotic Dis.*, 11, 8: 1209-1211.

Wahab T., Edvinsson B., Palm D., Lindh J. J. (2010): Comparison of the AF146527 and B1 repeated elements, two real-time PCR targets used for detection of Toxoplasma gondii. *Clin. Microbiol.*, 48, 2: 591-592.

Yera H., Filisetti D., Bastien P., Ancelle T., Thulliez P., Delhaes L. (2009): Multicenter comparative evaluation of five commercial methods for toxoplasma DNA extraction from amniotic fluid. *J. Clin. Microbiol.*, 47, 12: 3881-3886.

INDEX

B

C

D

E

F

G

H

I

M

Q

R

S

T

U

V

W

Y

Z